ABSOLUTE BEGINNER'S GUIDE

TO

Coaching Youth Baseball

Tom Hanlon

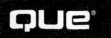

800 East 96th Street
Indianapolis, Indiana 46240

Absolute Beginner's Guide to Coaching Youth Baseball

Copyright © 2005 by Que Publishing

International Standard Book Number: 0-7897-3357-9

Library of Congress Catalog Card Number: 2004118018

Printed in the United States of America

This product is printed digitally on demand.

Trademarks

Warning and Disclaimer

Bulk Sales

Que Publishing offers excellent discounts on this book when ordered in quantity for bulk purchases or special sales. For more information, please contact

U.S. Corporate and Government Sales
1-800-382-3419
corpsales@pearsontechgroup.com

For sales outside the United States, please contact

International Sales
international@pearsoned.com

Publisher
Paul Boger

Executive Editor
Jeff Riley

Development Editor
Steve Rowe

Managing Editor
Charlotte Clapp

Project Editor
Dan Knott

Production Editor
Megan Wade

Indexer
Chris Barrick

Proofreader
Andrew Beaster

Technical Editor
Pat O'Neil

Publishing Coordinator
Pamalee Nelson

Interior Designer
Anne Jones

Cover Designer
Dan Armstrong

Page Layout
Susan Geiselman

Illustrations
Laura Robbins

Graphics
Tammy Graham

Contents at a Glance

Table of Contents

About the Author

Tom Hanlon has written more than 30 books, most in the areas of sports, coaching, and physical activity. His first love in sports is baseball, although you wouldn't know it by the way he plays softball. Hanlon lives in Champaign, Illinois, with his wife, Janet, and children, Tessa (an expert gymnast) and Trevor (whose goal is to play shortstop for the St. Louis Cardinals when he grows up).

Dedication

To Janet, for your undying love. And to all the youth baseball coaches who volunteer their time to teach kids the game and to facilitate those who dream of one day playing in the Major Leagues.

Acknowledgments

Many people used their talents to make this book happen. First and foremost, **Jeff Riley**, executive editor, paved the way for this book, inviting me to write it and getting it approved. I go back a long way with Jeff, although I normally don't admit that in public.

Steve Rowe, developmental editor, provided consistently excellent advice in shaping the content, in making the book as useful and practical as possible, and in managing all the details and tasks that go into developing a book.

Dan Knott, project editor and general baseball enthusiast, guided the project through to completion with skill, grace, and élan (read: he kept me on task).

Megan Wade lent her considerable talents as a copy editor, cleaning up and tightening the copy.

And **Patrick O'Neil**, head baseball coach for Brownsburg High School in Indiana, provided his expertise throughout the project and created the games and drills in Chapter 11.

We Want to Hear from You!

As the reader of this book, *you* are our most important critic and commentator. We value your opinion and want to know what we're doing right, what we could do better, what areas you'd like to see us publish in, and any other words of wisdom you're willing to pass our way.

As an executive editor for Que Publishing, I welcome your comments. You can email or write me directly to let me know what you did or didn't like about this book—as well as what we can do to make our books better.

Please note that I cannot help you with technical problems related to the topic of this book. We do have a User Services group, however, where I will forward specific technical questions related to the book.

When you write, please be sure to include this book's title and author as well as your name, email address, and phone number. I will carefully review your comments and share them with the author and editors who worked on the book.

Email: feedback@quepublishing.com

Mail: Jeff Riley
Executive Editor
Que Publishing
800 East 96th Street
Indianapolis, IN 46240 USA

For more information about this book or another Que title, visit our website at www.quepublishing.com. Type the ISBN (excluding hyphens) or the title of a book in the Search field to find the page you're looking for.

We Want to Hear from You!

As the reader of this book, *you* are our most important critic and commentator. We value your opinion and want to know what we're doing right, what we could do better, what areas you'd like to see us publish in, and any other words of wisdom you're willing to pass our way.

As an executive editor for Que Publishing, I welcome your comments. You can email or write me directly to let me know what you did or didn't like about this book—as well as what we can do to make our books better.

Please note that I cannot help you with technical problems related to the topic of this book. We do have a User Services group, however, where I will forward specific technical questions related to the book.

When you write, please be sure to include this book's title and author as well as your name, email address, and phone number. I will carefully review your comments and share them with the author and editors who worked on the book.

Email: feedback@quepublishing.com

Mail: Jeff Riley
Executive Editor
Que Publishing
800 East 96th Street
Indianapolis, IN 46240 USA

For more information about this book or another Que title, visit our website at www.quepublishing.com. Type the ISBN (excluding hyphens) or the title of a book in the Search field to find the page you're looking for.

INTRODUCTION

It all began so innocently.

Just as the youth baseball league administrator asked for a volunteer to coach your son's team, you scratched the top of your head. All the other parents were studying, with sudden keen interest, their thumbnails or shoelaces. No eyes, except yours, were looking forward.

The administrator saw her chance.

"Excellent! We have a new coach!"

To your astonishment, you saw that she was pointing directly at you. Parents, with relieved looks on their faces, turned to look at you. Some smirked. A few chuckled. All were joyful.

"Relax," one parent said. "The season doesn't start till next week."

"My kid's a slugger. You ought to see him smack that ball. He always bats cleanup," another parent said as he gave you a good view of the bulldog tattooed on his bicep.

"My son plays center field," another parent added, as if he bought his son the position from Major League Baseball, which had granted the boy sole rights to play center field on your team.

"I never knew you could coach, Dad," your son said as you walked to your car.

"Sure I can coach," you said. "How difficult can it be?" You hoped you at least *sounded* convincing.

Every spring, all across America, youth baseball leagues swing into action. Every year, thousands upon thousands of new coaches are tabbed to guide the players. The majority of those coaches have little or no experience coaching.

If you are one of those coaches, this book is for you. It is intended primarily for coaches of players from 6 to 12 years old, but it is applicable to coaches of older players as well. Use it as your rudder to guide you through your season. Use this book to

- Understand your role, and know what to expect, as a coach.
- Know the keys to being a good coach.
- Realize why kids play sports and consider how this should affect your approach to coaching.
- Bone up on the basic rules of baseball and learn how to impart those rules to your players.

- Provide for kids' safety and respond to emergency situations.
- Learn the general principles of teaching skills and tactics.
- Teach individual skills and team tactics.
- Coach effectively during games.
- Make the sport experience a meaningful and enjoyable one for the kids.
- Communicate effectively with parents, league administrators, umpires, and players.
- Form positive alliances with parents, involving them in various ways.
- Plan for your season and your practices.
- Discover the keys to conducting productive practices.
- Celebrate victories and learn from defeats.
- Keep it all in perspective.

This guide presents the foundational concepts that effective coaches follow, and it shows you, step-by-step, how to incorporate those concepts, plan your season, and conduct your practices. It provides many forms you will need, including sample and blank season and practice plans, a sample letter to parents, an injury report, an emergency information card, and a season evaluation form. It has games and drills you can use to teach your players the skills and tactics they need to know. It details how to execute the fundamental skills and tactics, so you will know what to teach— and it lays out *how* to teach. It is also replete with practical tips that will help your season be a success.

How This Book Is Organized

This book is organized in two parts. Part I, "Coaching Basics," provides guidance in a number of areas, including your basic approach to coaching, communication keys, safety principles, and practice planning. Part II, "Skills and Tactics," delves into the specifics of the skills and tactics your players will need to learn, ending with an entire chapter devoted to games and drills you can use to teach those skills and tactics.

Following Part II are six appendixes you should find useful. This material includes a sample letter to parents, a medical emergency form, an injury report, blank season and practice plans you can use for your own planning, and a season evaluation form you can use at the end of your season.

Special Elements

Throughout the book you will find the following special elements:

caution

Cautions give you a loud "Heads up!" regarding issues or situations you want to avoid. These point out pitfalls, potential safety hazards, and any other items that could pose trouble to you or your team.

note

This is a note element. Notes give you relevant information that doesn't necessarily fit in the text flow.

tip

Tips are given to help you do something more efficiently or to give you the "inside" view on how to accomplish something related to coaching baseball.

warning

Warnings are always safety-related, and are used with issues or situations of more serious consequence than those associated with cautions.

PART 1

COACHING BASICS

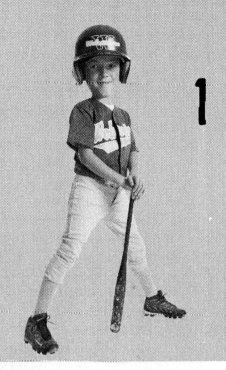

1

YOUR COACHING APPROACH

So you're a coach! Excellent. Most likely, you have a week or so to prepare for your first practice. But it's not time to jump into practice planning yet. Just as you will want your players to develop their fundamental skills first, you need to develop your basic coaching approach. Consider this chapter as your own personal spring training. It provides the foundation for you to build upon.

Your Coaching Philosophy

When Charles Dickens began *A Tale of Two Cities* with "It was the best of times, it was the worst of times, it was the season of Light, it was the season of Darkness...," he wasn't describing the typical youth league season, but he could have been.

Competition can bring out the best in us, and it can bring out the worst in us. You've read the stories of coaches fighting with other coaches or with 16-year-old umpires. You've probably witnessed parents in the bleachers screaming at the umpires or at opposing players—or at their own kids. It doesn't happen all the time, but it happens often enough, even at the earliest levels of competition.

And it happens because of an overemphasis on winning. Our society places a premium on winning, and generally on winning at all costs. "Just win, baby," was the motto coined by Oakland Raiders owner Al Davis. This motto is fine at the professional level. It is *not* fine at the youth level. Why? Because when your focus is solely on winning, it comes at the expense of the kids you coach.

When your primary goal is to have an undefeated season or to win your league title, what happens? Every decision you make is based on whether it will help you win. So, you play Colin, Seth, and Max, your least-skilled players, as little as your league rules allow. You pinch-hit for them so you can add to your 5-run lead. You place Kendra in right field, and instruct your swift and sure-handed center fielder, Zach, to field anything he can get his hands on, even if it's Kendra's ball. You tell Sam, who is small, to scrunch down at the plate and to take the first two strikes, in hopes of drawing a walk.

At the professional level, at the collegiate and high school levels, and even at upper youth levels, there's nothing wrong with this. At the lower youth levels, certainly at ages 6–12, plenty is wrong with it.

That overemphasis on winning comes at the cost of the kids' development, and of their love for the game. It results in low morale when players don't win enough games to meet your, or their parents', expectations. It certainly discourages the lesser-skilled players, who thought they were going to play a game but find that their main duty is to warm the bench and cheer on their teammates. It sends the message to kids that if they don't win, they have failed in their mission.

But their mission when they are 6–12 years old is to learn the game, to acquire and improve their skills, to gain in their understanding of the rules

tip

Remember, the only way kids are going to improve their skills is by receiving good instruction and playing the game. At this level, that's your mission: to give everyone solid instruction and playing experience.

and tactics. It is not to pummel the opponent, to make a name for themselves in the local media, to win every title in sight.

Your approach, then, should be to develop the whole player in these ways: physically, mentally, emotionally, and socially.

Physical Development

It's your task as a coach to help your players acquire and develop the physical skills they need to perform. You need to teach them the basics: batting, pitching, fielding, throwing, running the bases, and so on.

In Chapter 6, "Player Development," you'll learn how to teach skills and tactics, and Chapters 9 and 10 are devoted to the correct execution of the skills and tactics you will be teaching, so you'll know step-by-step how to demonstrate proper execution.

Players' physical development is one of the obvious duties of a coach, and one that takes preeminence in practice. But practices and games can be used to develop players in other ways as well, including their mental development.

Mental Development

There's a player on third base with one out. The batter lifts a fly ball to center field. The player on third takes off and crosses home plate at about the same time the center fielder catches the ball. The offensive coach is shouting at his player to return to third base. The defensive coach is shouting at her center fielder to throw the ball to the third baseman, who is looking at a kid flying a kite a little ways away. The center fielder tosses the ball to the shortstop, who flips it to the pitcher. As the defensive coach tells her players, for the fifteenth time, "He didn't tag up!" the pitcher throws it to his catcher, thinking maybe that's what his coach wants him to do. "Step on the plate!" the pitcher shouts as the catcher catches the toss. But the catcher knows better: He lofts a throw to the third baseman, only the ball goes over his head and is retrieved by the left fielder, who, a little uncertain at first, finally jogs over to third base and steps on it. The defensive coach collapses to her knees in joy, and then makes a note—as does the opposing coach—to teach her players the tag-up rule at their next practice.

Especially at the youth level, kids won't know all the rules and they won't know many—if any—of the strategies of the game. If you teach skills in the context of how your players will use them in a game and tell them why they need to know how to do the skill, chances are they will retain the *why* part. Also be aware that they might not understand these items the first few times you tell them, but as you continue to teach and remind them, it should sink in.

One of the greatest joys of coaching is seeing that your players know what to do in game situations. For example, they understand when it's a force situation or a tag situation; they understand they can run on any ball hit with two outs; they understand they have to tag up on a fly ball with less than two outs. The outfielders know which base to throw to, and the infielders know where to line up to cut off a throw from the outfield.

This won't happen all at once, and much of it might not happen at all at the youngest levels. But if you clearly and simply explain the basic tactics and help them understand the game and how to respond to various situations, their mental development is fun to watch. The mark of a good team, especially at the youth level, is not that they execute every play perfectly, but that they know what they should be trying to do in each situation.

Emotional Development

Each player is a unique person. Some players are outgoing; some are reserved. Some are excitable, and some laid-back. Some are jokers; some are serious. Some have the attention span of a gnat; others soak in most of what you say.

As a coach it is crucial that you understand that any one approach won't work the same with each child. Ben might be fine with some gentle kidding, whereas Alex might be bothered by the same kidding. Get to know your players as best you can in the first few weeks, and instruct and encourage them in the ways that will help them be ready and eager to learn and to play.

Remember that games produce situations that can become quite emotional for players (not to mention coaches!). Some players will be disconsolate after a loss; others won't be bothered at all. Help keep your players on an even keel. We talk more about how to do so in Chapter 7, "Game Time!"

Social Development

Baseball is great for social development. It takes a team effort to win. Players must rely on each other, pull for each other, and learn how to play with each other as they strive to win.

Use teachable moments to emphasize the team aspect of baseball. Such moments include a force out at second base, a cutoff play on a fly ball, and a sacrifice bunt. All involve teammates and all are executed for the good of the team.

Reinforce team unity in practices and at games. Don't treat "star" players differently. Look to enfold "fringe" players, those who are quiet or lesser-skilled and who might otherwise go unnoticed, in all team aspects. Also, be sure to emphasize the importance of everyone's contributions and point out those contributions when they happen.

Some Final Thoughts on Your Coaching Philosophy

Winning is a worthy goal, and one you should pursue as a team. However, as a youth baseball coach, winning cannot be the ultimate goal because the physical, mental, emotional, and social development of each player should be your ultimate goal.

When you develop your players' physical talents and mental abilities, you are putting them in a position to win. Teach them the game and its rules and tactics so they will be prepared to perform to the best of their abilities and knowledge. Encourage your players; let them know it's all right to make mistakes, and to learn from those mistakes.

When you focus on developing the whole player, that doesn't mean you're necessarily going to win your league or have a high winning percentage. It means you're keeping winning in its proper place—as a byproduct of sound player development, keeping each child's best interests at heart.

Sound difficult? It's not, if you develop the attributes of a good coach.

10 Attributes of a Good Coach

Just as your players are unique individuals, so are coaches. Maybe you're an extrovert; maybe you're an introvert. Maybe you're in a leadership position at work and are used to supervising people; maybe you have no supervisory experience at all. Regardless of your background, you can be an excellent youth baseball coach if you develop the following 10 attributes:

- Take your role seriously—but not *too* seriously.
- Be comfortable with being in charge.
- Be dependable and stable.
- Be patient.
- Be flexible.
- Enjoy getting to know your players.
- Desire to help kids learn and grow.
- Be an encourager.
- Be willing to learn.
- Have a sense of humor.

Let's take a brief look at each attribute.

Take Your Role Seriously

Now that you have volunteered to coach, commit yourself to the time and energy it will take to coach. Showing up on time at the practice field or for the game is not enough. Show up prepared to conduct the practice, prepared to coach your players during the game, and ready to instruct and supervise your players. Your role is to teach your players how to play baseball. They're looking to learn from you.

On the other hand, keep things in their proper perspective. These are games, learning experiences—and intended to be *fun* learning experiences—for kids who are 6– to 12 years old. Their baseball experience generally *is* fun, win or lose, unless it is tarnished by overzealous coaches or parents who place such great emphasis on winning that all the fun drains out of the game.

Keep the fun in the game. Keep the kids' best interests at heart. Relax; take a deep breath; enjoy the sunshine; and focus on the task at hand, such as how to field a ground ball, which base to throw to, or how to swing the bat.

Use your players as a guide. If they look tense or are unusually quiet at practice, or if they're avoiding your look, they're probably taking their cues from you, and you better lighten up your approach. On the other hand, if they're cracking jokes and goofing off and aren't focusing on the task at hand, you need to gain control. You'll learn some tips on how to do so in Chapter 5, "Practice Plans."

Ultimately what you're after is a steady pace at practice where learning and fun are synonymous and ongoing.

Be Comfortable with Being in Charge

Every child will be looking to you for instruction. You have to be comfortable with being the leader, the teacher, and the resident expert who knows how to instruct and conduct effective practices. There's a fine line between having fun at practice and simply goofing off. You need to know what your goal is in each practice, and you need to steer your kids in that direction while maintaining an open and friendly atmosphere within that context.

If you're not comfortable being in charge and are unable to set the proper tone for practice, one of two things happens: either the practice crumbles into chaos and nothing is learned as kids misbehave and don't pay attention, or you overreact to a little goofing off and rule with severe authority.

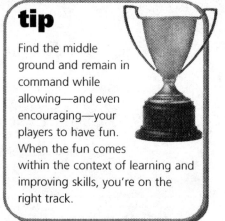

tip

Find the middle ground and remain in command while allowing—and even encouraging—your players to have fun. When the fun comes within the context of learning and improving skills, you're on the right track.

Be Dependable and Stable

Be on time at every practice and game, and be there ready to execute your plan. If you can't make a game or practice, alert your assistant coach or a parent who is willing and able to take over.

The kids are counting on you. When they know they can rely on you to be there and be ready, that lets them focus on learning, practicing, and performing. When the kids know that you respond evenly and fairly in all situations, they feel free to practice without worrying about how you might respond to an error or a strikeout. Coaches who are dependable and stable create a healthy learning environment for their players.

Be Patient

If you're a parent, you know the value of patience. It can be difficult enough raising a couple of young kids. When you have 15 youngsters at your charge, patience is at a premium.

They won't pay attention to your every word. They won't always understand your instruction on the first, or second or third, try. They will make the same types of errors over and over again. They will ask you goofy questions and act, well, like the kids they are. They will, in short, try your patience. If you don't have a lot, here's your chance to develop this virtue.

Don't expect perfection, either in game-time performance or practice field behavior. Let the kids know what you expect of them, in terms of their behavior and their listening to your directives. Also keep in mind what the goal is for the day, whether you're at a practice or a game, and steer the ship in that direction. When you guide your players with patient resolve, your practices will be more effective.

Don't mistake being patient with letting your players do whatever they want to do. Don't tolerate inappropriate words or actions. Step in and correct players in these situations. Just remember to be patient as they strive to learn how to hit, field, throw, pitch, and run the bases.

caution

Some parents might try your patience, too. You'll learn ways to communicate with them and tips for maintaining your cool as you do so in Chapter 3, "Communication Keys."

Be Flexible

Being flexible is another hallmark of a good coach. You might have worked out your season plan, in terms of what you want to teach and when you want to teach it, but you might have to adjust that schedule if the kids haven't picked up the requisite skills yet. For example, it's no use teaching your 10-year-olds how to execute a double play if they are having trouble simply fielding ground balls and making throws to first.

You have to constantly assess how your players are doing, what they need to learn next, and what they have been able to master at least well enough to move on to something new. It's good to work out a season plan in advance; just be ready to adjust that plan along the way.

Enjoy Getting to Know Your Players

Hopefully you enjoy being around kids, or you wouldn't have volunteered to coach. The best coaches appreciate kids for who they are and want to help them develop their skills and learn a sport. These coaches understand that their players are full-fledged children, not miniature adults. And these coaches enjoy being around their players. They can see the game from their players' perspectives while maintaining their adult view and their authority as a coach. They appreciate each child for his own unique personality and skills.

With that in mind, realize that the approach that works with Justin, who is effusive and outgoing, might not work with Sam, who is quiet and reflective. Learn to communicate with players on an individual level. Pay attention to what each player responds best to, and develop a rapport with each child that will help him learn and grow best.

That doesn't mean you should change your personality to suit each player. It means you should be aware of each child's distinct personality and relate to him as an individual.

Getting to know your players on an individual level is one of the joys of coaching. By doing so, you can tune into their needs as players and more readily help them develop their skills.

Desire to Help Kids Learn and Grow

There are two outs, late in a tight ballgame, with runners at second and third. Michael, your third baseman, fields a ground ball and steps on third, believing he's forced out the runner on second. The run scores and everyone is safe. Needless to say, this can be frustrating. But, you have two choices at this point:

- First, you could chew Michael out in front of the other players for his bone-headed play, shouting that you've gone over and over what a force out is and how he should know this by now, adding that he should have thrown to first base.

▨ Second, you could calmly remind Michael of the force-out rule and tell him the next time he's in that situation to make the play at first. Then tell him to let it go, give him some sincere encouragement, and turn your attention to the next hitter.

Hopefully, you would choose the latter. You're more likely to do so if your focus is on helping the players learn and grow. This is really what coaching is all about at the youth level. It's very satisfying to watch your players acquire new skills, learn the game's tactics, and be able to execute plays more consistently. These things happen when your central desire as a coach is to help them learn and grow.

Be an Encourager

Good instruction is the seed and encouragement is the water that helps the seed grow. Your players need your encouragement as they attempt to learn the physical and mental skills it takes to play baseball. You'll learn more about specific ways to encourage your players in Chapter 3.

Be Willing to Learn

Just as your players will be learning throughout the season how to play the game, you'll be learning how to coach. There are many ways you can learn:

▨ **Through this book**—Use this guide to shape your approach to coaching and to formulate your season and practice plans.

▨ **Through your own experience**—Know that you'll make some mistakes along the way. That's okay. Be willing to learn from your mistakes. You'll discover, through experience, what works for you and what doesn't. You might also find that what works well for you this year might not work as well next year with different players.

▨ **Through observing other coaches**—You can learn from both good and bad coaches. What sets good coaches apart from ones who aren't so good? How do they communicate with their players, and *what* do they communicate? How do they behave on the bench or in the dugout? How do they relate with umpires, and what kind of coaching do they do during the game? How do their players conduct themselves during and after the game? You can learn a lot through observation. Put to use what works for you, and model yourself after competent and caring coaches.

▨ **Through coaching clinics**—If your league offers a coaching clinic, attend it. If not, keep your eye out for coaching clinics in your area. You can often pick up some pointers and make helpful contacts at these clinics.

Most importantly, be willing to learn to coach. Many former players rely solely on their playing experience to inform their coaching. With that same thinking, you might assume that because you've had experience sitting in a dentist's chair and having a tooth drilled, you are qualified to pick up a dentist's drill and go to work in someone's mouth.

Playing and coaching call on a different set of skills. Having playing experience can help you as a coach in many ways, but it doesn't take the place of knowing how to coach. This book will help you develop your coaching skills.

Have a Sense of Humor

Enjoy your time as a coach. Baseball is meant to be fun. Your intent as a coach shouldn't be to "entertain the troops," but there's nothing wrong with a little natural levity. It's okay to laugh and joke with your players; you can do this while still moving forward with your instruction.

Just make sure your humor doesn't come at the expense of someone else—even an opponent. Don't make fun of someone's mistake, but do enjoy lighthearted moments as they come up.

Don't use humor when kids need instruction, but do use it to diffuse tension. For example, if Jimmy is about to bat with the bases loaded, facing a tough, hard-throwing pitcher, and he asks what he should do, don't say, "How about a grand slam? We could use four runs." Jimmy's not asking for a joke, but for a little help. He'd be better-served if you told him, "Just stay with the pitch and try to drive it. Don't try to pull it. If he goes outside on you, go to right field. Just meet the ball with a nice, level swing."

caution

Having fun and being friendly with the kids doesn't mean you should try to be best buds with them. They're not looking for a new friend; they're looking for a coach to help them learn the game.

10 Keys to Being a Good Coach

We've just gone over the attributes of a good coach. If you have those attributes, or can develop them, you're on your way to being a good coach. But some other key elements to coaching extend beyond these basic characteristics. When you exhibit the traits we talked about in the previous section and possess the 10 keys we present in this section, you'll excel.

What are the keys to good coaching? To be a good baseball coach, you must

- Know the basics of the sport.
- Plan for your season and practices.

- Conduct effective practices.
- Teach skills and tactics.
- Correct players in a way that helps them improve.
- Teach and model good sporting behavior.
- Provide for safety.
- Communicate effectively with players, parents, umpires, and league administrators.
- Coach effectively during games.
- Know what constitutes success in youth baseball.

Let's look at each of these keys in a little more depth.

Know the Basics of the Sport

You can't teach what you don't know. You need to be prepared to teach your players the basic rules, the skills, and the tactics of baseball. Especially at the younger ages, this information is quite basic, but that doesn't mean you automatically know all you need to know.

The next chapter covers the basic rules and Chapters 9 and 10 cover the skills and tactics you need to know and teach. Be sure you know the rules, skills, and tactics before your season begins.

Plan for Your Season and Practices

You can know all you need to know about the rules, skills, and tactics, but if you don't have a game plan for when and how to teach them, you—and, more importantly, your players—will be in trouble.

Planning doesn't mean thinking about a drill you might run that day as you drive to practice. It means considering the big picture for the entire season and breaking that picture down into individual practice plans so you're prepared for every practice. You'll learn how to create season and practice plans in Chapter 5.

Conduct Effective Practices

When you have a practice plan in hand, you are on your way to conducting an effective practice. But, there's a big difference between having a plan and being able to execute it. Two coaches could have the exact same practice plan, and the experiences could be vastly different for their players depending on how the coaches execute that plan. In Chapter 5 you'll learn the keys to conducting effective practices.

Teach Skills and Tactics

This, of course, is one of your primary duties. Your ability to teach skills and tactics will significantly impact your players' development. Remember, the abilities to *perform* and to *teach* are different abilities. So, if you've played before, don't assume your playing experience will make you a great teacher.

Rather, learn how to be an effective teacher. In Chapter 6 you'll learn the keys to teaching skills and tactics.

Correct Players in a Way That Helps Them Improve

If one of your players makes the same mistake repeatedly, it might be he's simply unable to perform the skill yet—or it might be you haven't helped him understand *how* to correct his error. Part of being an effective teacher is being able to observe your players' performances, detect mechanical and tactical errors, and help them correct those errors. In Chapter 6, you'll learn how to detect and correct errors and help your players improve their skills.

Teach and Model Good Sporting Behavior

Your players will take their cues from you, not only on how to play the game, but also in how to behave at games. Behave responsibly and treat all involved with respect. Leave the arguing and gamesmanship for major league managers. You'll learn more on modeling good behavior in Chapter 7.

Provide for Players' Safety

This is one of your most important duties. You'll need to know how to conduct safe practices and how to respond to injuries when they occur. Chapter 4, "Safety Principles," is devoted to this topic.

Communicate Effectively

You'll do a lot of communicating as a coach, primarily with your players, but also with their parents, umpires, other coaches, and league administrators. You might know exactly how to field a ground ball, but if you don't know how to communicate how to do so, your players probably won't understand the mechanics involved. Chapter 3 explains how to communicate effectively—and what needs to be communicated and to whom—in a variety of situations.

Coach Effectively During Games

There's a difference between coaching at practice and coaching during games. The goals are different, and what you communicate is different. You'll learn about those differences, and the keys to coaching effectively during games, in Chapter 7.

Know What Success Is

By now you should have the idea that success at the youth level isn't based on your winning percentage. Rather, it's based on your ability to develop your players' skills and help them maintain their enthusiasm for the game, and on many other factors. Winning is an important and worthy goal, but you can have a successful season no matter what your record is. In Chapter 8, "Ingredients of a Successful Season," you'll learn what makes a season *truly* successful, and you'll also learn how to gauge your success.

Final Thoughts on the Keys to Being a Good Coach

When you use these 10 keys as the foundation of your coaching, you'll be successful. In fact, learning how to use these keys is what the rest of Part I, "Coaching Basics," is all about.

What to Expect As a Coach

The dream of youth league coaches goes something like this:

- All their players show up on time for every practice.
- The players pay attention every minute.
- The players soak in the instruction and acquire the physical skills and tactical knowledge with ease.
- The players perform like seasoned veterans from game 1.
- The parents are enthusiastic, supportive, and appreciative of the coach's efforts and ability to bring the team together.
- After winning the league championship, the players are somehow able to hoist the coach up on their scrawny shoulders and the parents roar their approval.
- To cap everything off, one rich parent throws a victory party at an expensive steak house, and during the party the teary-eyed parents come by, one by one, to thank the coach for making such a difference in their son's or daughter's life.

Conversely, the nightmare of youth league coaches goes something like this:

- You have to call all your players the night before the first practice because the league switched your practice field at the last moment.
- Not all the players assigned to your team show up for the first practice.
- The time you meant to take to plan for the season and the first practice evaporated, and you feel rushed and unprepared.
- About half the kids on your team have never played baseball before.
- A couple of kids are uncooperative.
- Another kid sprains his ankle in the first practice.
- At the first game, you have your lineup made out, but three players don't show up until the second inning, so you have to rearrange everything at the last moment.
- You find that two fathers are more than willing to shout helpful coaching tips to you, while a mother sits behind home plate and critiques the umpire.
- After the game, a couple of parents complain about what position you played their child in, or where you batted her in the batting order.
- Rain wipes out three games.
- Your calls to the league administrator are never returned.

Hopefully that nightmare won't be your reality. But the point is this: Be prepared for anything. Know that mundane, tedious, and sometimes bothersome things will infiltrate your season.

Expect to be tested, in some ways by your players, in others by their parents. Expect the umpiring to be less than perfect. Expect a few rainouts and a few hastily scheduled makeup dates at inopportune times. Expect your players to make mistakes, and expect some of them to be upset by those mistakes. Expect some parents to be very supportive, others to be seemingly nonexistent, and a few to present challenging situations. Expect the unexpected, and know that not all things will go according to your plan.

Keep your focus on what's best for the kids, and base all your decisions on that. That's why it's so important to develop the attributes of a good coach. When you are patient, flexible, dependable, and comfortable with being in charge, you can handle any situation that comes your way.

What Is Expected of *You* As a Coach

What is expected of you is summed up in the keys to good coaching:

- You are expected to know the basics of baseball, its rules, its strategies, and the skills involved.

- You are expected to be prepared to coach—to plan for the season and for practices—so that there is a logical cohesiveness to your instruction, a purpose for each practice, and a sense of moving forward throughout the season, with the players always learning and always improving.

- You are expected to be able to teach the skills and tactics of baseball, explain when and how the skill or tactic is used, and demonstrate how to execute it. (If you are unable to adequately demonstrate it, you can use an assistant coach or a volunteer parent to do so.)

- You are expected to observe your players as they practice the skills and tactics to detect what they are doing incorrectly and to help them make corrections.

- You are expected to model good sporting behavior; communicate appropriately with players, parents, umpires, and the opposition; and show respect for all involved.

- You are expected to teach your players how to win with class without rubbing it in or taunting their opponents, and how to lose with dignity, learning from the loss and making neither a win nor a loss bigger than it is.

- You are expected to conduct practices as safely as possible, providing direct supervision at all times, conducting drills and games that are safe, warning players about inherent dangers, and instituting team rules concerning swinging bats and throwing balls that promote safety.

- You are expected to know how to coach during games, doing what's appropriate and best for your players' development and conducting yourself appropriately.

- Finally, you are expected to keep in mind what constitutes success in youth baseball. You are striving to win your games, of course, but far greater than that, you are giving your players opportunities to develop their skills, to have fun, to compete, to play together as a team, and to get the most of their abilities. They are there to grow, learn, and develop, and that development is your main task.

Now, not all parents or players will have these expectations. Some will be focused only on winning and become frustrated if your coaching decisions don't reflect the same outlook. In Chapter 3 you'll learn when and how to communicate with players and parents who have these expectations.

It's important that you keep these expectations in mind throughout the season. They will act as your rudder, guiding you through any choppy waters you might experience.

Equipment and Insurance

Check with your league regarding equipment they issue each team and insurance they might carry. In many cases, the league provides batting helmets, bats, balls, and catcher's equipment for each team, and it's your responsibility to keep and maintain the equipment and return it at season's end.

In addition, you should have a scorebook for your games. You'll learn the basics of scorekeeping in Chapter 7.

In some cases, insurance is provided through a coaching certification program or a league; in other cases, it's not provided. Some leagues carry insurance policies that cover all teams and participants involved, including coaches and umpires. If insurance is an important issue for you, talk to your league administrator about it.

Last, But Not Least: Why Kids Play Baseball

Kids play baseball for a lot of reasons. Many have grand dreams of being the next Barry Bonds, Alex Rodriguez, Albert Pujols, Roger Clemens, or whoever their favorite player is.

Some play for negative reasons, such as their parents pushing them into it. Their father might be trying to relive his faded dreams of stardom. Or, they might have chosen baseball over a less desirable activity, such as taking tuba lessons.

But the overwhelming majority play for positive reasons. Those reasons are

- They want to have fun.
- They want to hang out with their friends.
- They want to develop their abilities.
- They like the excitement of sports.
- They want to be part of a winning effort.

That order is not random; it reflects the most common responses kids give when they are asked for the main reasons they play baseball.

Notice that *fun* is at the top of the list, and *winning* is at the bottom. Winning is important to them, but not nearly as important as it is to have fun and be with their friends.

What does this mean for you? It means you should focus on fun and development throughout the season and that you should strive to win, but not at the expense of fun and development. It's that simple. And you'll be amazed at how well your players perform when they're having fun and developing their skills.

THE ABSOLUTE MINIMUM

This chapter introduced you to the basic concepts of coaching baseball. You learned about your coaching approach, the attributes of a good coach, the keys to being a good coach, what you should expect as a coach, what is expected of you as a coach, and why kids play baseball. Keep these points in mind:

- Base your coaching approach on players' fun and development. Always keep their overall development in mind.
- Keep the attributes of a good coach front and center. When you approach your coaching with these traits in mind, you are bound to be successful.
- Plan your practices. Learn how to teach skills and tactics and how to correct mistakes.
- Expect the unexpected, and be guided by your coaching approach in all situations.
- Live up to your own expectations, based on the keys to good coaching.
- Understand that kids play baseball to have fun, to be with their friends, and to develop their skills.

Coaching with these things in mind will help you plan and implement a fun and constructive baseball season that produces enjoyment and plenty of learning!

2

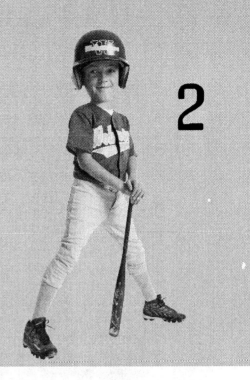

RULES OF THE GAME

Baseball has some basic rules that even the most casual fan knows:

- Three strikes and you're out.
- Three outs in each half inning.
- Catch a ball in the air and the batter's out.
- Four balls and the batter is awarded first base.
- A baserunner on first has to touch second on his way to third, rather than taking a shortcut around the pitcher's mound. (Plenty of youthful runners have tried the shortcut route, to no avail.)
- No more than one runner can occupy a base at the same time. (Seems easy enough, but three Brooklyn Dodgers once occupied third base at the same time, and two of them were tagged out—and that's the *major* leagues!)

There are a host of rules your players need to be aware of, and as their coach, it's your duty to teach them those rules. What's a force out, and what does that mean for the runner and the fielder? When is a tag play called for, and what does *that* mean for the baserunners and fielders? What's the tag-up rule mean, and when does it apply? What about the infield fly rule?

Here are just some of the questions you'll need to know the answers to: Can batters bunt? Are baserunners allowed to lead off? Are they allowed to steal? If so, at what point can they take off? How many innings can your pitchers pitch per game and per week? What are the substitution rules? Is a designated hitter allowed?

In addition to the basic rules, you have to know the modified rules of your league and relay those modifications to your players. Many rules are modified to make the game more appropriate for younger players. For example, some leagues have modified rules for balls and strikes, for running the bases, and for the number of players allowed on the field. If you're at younger levels, you might be playing coach-pitch or machine-pitch. Fields are proportioned to the age and size of the players—pitching distances, base paths, and fences are shortened for younger players and gradually become longer and farther as the players grow older. Some leagues instill time limits on games, and many have a 10-run rule after four innings, meaning if one team is ahead by 10 runs after the trailing team has batted in the fourth inning, the game is over. Check with your league administrator to learn which modified rules your league has in place.

While your primary duty is to teach your players the skills they need to perform well, they need to understand the context within which they'll perform those skills, and the rules provide part of that context.

In this chapter, then, you'll learn about the basic rules so you can prepare your players to know what to do with the ball on defense and what to do on the base paths.

Basic Youth Baseball Rules

The following is meant to be a primer for the basics, not the final word on every rule in complete detail. The rules in this section are divided into seven categories:

- Field
- Equipment
- Players
- Pitching
- Hitting
- Fielding
- Baserunning

note

Be sure to read the "Terms" section later in this chapter because many rules are explained there.

Field

Baseball is played on a field that has a home plate and first, second, and third bases (see Figure 2.1). In many leagues, a safety base is used at first base. This is a double base, with one base used by the first baseman in receiving throws from infielders and the other base (usually a different color) used by the batter/runner who is trying to beat out a hit. The double base decreases the likelihood of an injury resulting from the first baseman and batter/runner getting tangled up at the bag. After a runner has reached first base safely, he then uses the bag that is closest to second base—the one the first baseman uses.

FIGURE 2.1

A basic baseball field.

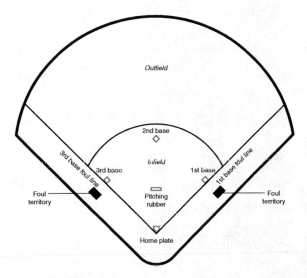

The *infield* is the portion of the field that contains the bases; the *outfield* is beyond the infield, bordered by the foul lines and fence. One foul line runs from home plate to first base and continues down the right field line, ending at the fence; the other foul line runs from home plate to third base and continues down the left field line, ending at the fence. The pitcher pitches from a pitching rubber in the middle of the infield, usually on a raised mound.

The pitching distance (the distance from the pitching rubber to home plate), the distance between bases, and the distance from home plate to the outfield fence are adjusted according to age. Typical distances are 46 feet for pitching, 60 feet between the bases, and 200 feet to the fence, but these can fluctuate between leagues and age groups within leagues.

Fair or Foul?

Here are a few rules concerning whether a ball is fair or foul:

▓ If a batted ball lands in fair territory in the infield but is not touched by a player and rolls foul before it passes either first base or third base, it is a foul ball. If it is touched by a fielder in fair territory and then rolls foul, it is a fair ball.

▓ If a batted ball is hit in the air and is fair as it passes over either first or third base, but initially touches down in foul territory without having been touched by a fielder, the ball is foul.

▓ If a ball is touching any part of the foul line, it is considered to be in fair territory.

▓ If a ball bounces over the outfield fence in fair territory, it's a ground-rule double and all runners, including the batter/runner, advance two bases.

Equipment

Baseball is played with balls, bats, gloves, helmets, and catcher's equipment. Check with your league for equipment specifications. Here are general parameters for equipment:

▓ **Balls**—Safety (softer) balls are used at younger levels. Standard size is 9"–9 1/4" in circumference, weighing 5–5 1/2 ounces.

▓ **Bats**—Leagues generally have rules regarding the minimum and maximum bat lengths. Bats are either aluminum or wood. Make sure your players use bats they can easily swing; sometimes smaller players choose bats that are too big or heavy, and they have trouble generating much bat speed.

tip

If players' gloves are new and stiff, suggest they treat their gloves with oil (specially made for baseball gloves and available in sporting goods stores). The oil softens and preserves the glove. The best way to store a glove when it's not being used is with a couple of baseballs in its pocket to preserve the shape.

▓ **Gloves**—At the youth level, gloves are similar except for the catcher's glove. There aren't any rules to concern yourself with here, but check to see that players have gloves that fit well. A loose-fitting or too-large glove makes fielding difficult.

▓ **Helmets**—Batting helmets are mandatory and are usually provided by the league. Batters, on-deck hitters, and baserunners must wear helmets. Make sure the helmet fits snugly on the player's head, that it doesn't flop around when he swings, and that it covers his ears.

■ **Catcher's equipment**—Catcher's equipment includes a face mask, a helmet, a chest protector, shinguards, and a catcher's glove (see Figure 2.2). Again, make sure the mask fits snugly over the player's face and that all the equipment fits well.

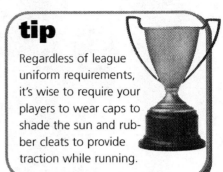

In addition to the equipment just mentioned, players are usually required to wear some type of uniform, ranging from a complete uniform with baseball socks, pants, jersey, cleats, and caps to team t-shirts and shorts.

Players

Normally there are nine players on the field (see Figure 2.3). The players are assigned numbers according to the position they play (these aren't their uniform numbers; the numbers correspond only to their position and are used to record fielding plays). The positions are

1 – Pitcher   6 – Shortstop
2 – Catcher   7 – Left fielder
3 – First baseman   8 – Center fielder
4 – Second baseman   9 – Right fielder
5 – Third baseman

FIGURE 2.2
A catcher in full equipment.

FIGURE 2.3
Player positions on the field.

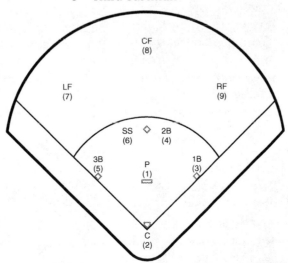

In some leagues for younger players, 10 players are allowed on the field. Generally, the 10th player plays in the outfield. Many leagues also allow a designated hitter; you'll read more about this in "Hitting Rules."

Also, check your league rules regarding substitutions. Some leagues have open substitution rules, where players can be subbed in and out as many times as you want; others have substitution limits.

Following are some tips for placing players in various positions:

- **Pitcher**—Pitching is one of the most difficult skills for youngsters to master. This is one position where you *don't* want to place every player because it can be humiliating for a child to walk batter after batter. Place kids on the mound who have strong and accurate arms (accuracy is more important than speed at this point). Don't allow them to try to throw curveballs or any other type of pitch that puts more strain on their arms than a fastball does.

- **Catcher**—This is another position that you should not place every player in. Many kids aren't comfortable catching pitches in a crouched position with a lot of equipment on and with a batter swinging a bat just a few feet away. Your best bet is to place sure-handed players behind the plate if they are comfortable catching pitches.

- **First baseman**—The first baseman needs sure hands because he will be called on to catch a lot of throws from infielders who field ground balls.

- **Second baseman**—The second baseman needs to be able to move laterally and field ground balls. Leg speed and arm strength

tip

At younger levels it's important for players to play at various positions. As they gain in experience, age, and skill, they can begin to focus on one or two positions. At least through age 9, though, move players around to give them experience at various positions.

caution

To reiterate what was previously mentioned about throwing curve balls, it is very important to encourage young players to stay away from throwing anything but fastballs. Players can hurt their arms, sometimes severely, at younger ages when throwing curveballs, screwballs, or other pitches that are not straight fastballs. Make parents aware of this, too. You don't want your kids to harm their careers early on!

note

You'll learn how to help players develop their pitching skills in Chapter 10, "Defensive Skills and Tactics."

are not as important as having a soft glove (meaning he can field ground balls) and an accurate throwing arm.

- **Third baseman**—The third baseman is called on to make longer throws, and thus arm strength is a necessity here. Third basemen also need to have quick reactions and a bit of fearlessness because sharply hit balls can reach them quickly.

- **Shortstop**—The shortstop is often the best fielder on the team, among the most sure-handed and with a strong, accurate arm.

- **Left fielder**—The left fielder, as do all the outfielders, benefits from being able to judge fly balls, knowing whether to break in or back on balls hit in his direction. Outfielders also benefit from having strong arms because their throws are often longer than those of infielders.

- **Center fielder**—Center field calls for the most speed because the center fielder covers more ground than the corner outfielders. Again, being able to effectively track the ball after it is hit and a good arm are keys to playing center field.

- **Right fielder**—Some coaches try to "hide" their weaker players in right field, but this doesn't make much sense because the right fielder gets a fair amount of action and needs to make the plays the same as the other outfielders. In fact, the right fielder should have a stronger arm than the left fielder because the right fielder has a longer throw to third base.

Some players are more suited to the infield, better able to field ground balls and make accurate throws to the proper base. Others are more suited to the outfield, where they can put their speed and ability to track balls—that is, their ability to judge where the ball is going to land, and run to that spot while keeping the ball in sight—to use.

Some coaches are tempted to play their strongest players only in what they consider the key positions: pitcher, catcher, shortstop, and center field. There are two thoughts to consider here: First, every position is key. All your players are going to be involved in the field. Second, players 9 years old or younger should not be pigeonholed into a certain position, either in trying to take advantage of their skills or in trying to hide their deficiencies. When they are 10, they can begin to focus on one or two positions, but before then, they should learn all or most of the positions. Remember, it's not all about *you* winning as a coach; it's all about *them* gaining experience, learning the game, and having fun as players.

Pitching Rules

At younger levels, players don't pitch; they either hit off a tee (T-ball) or are pitched to by coaches or pitching machines.

When players begin pitching (usually by age nine), many leagues have restrictions on how many innings per game and per week a player can pitch. Check with your league on this.

The strike zone is defined as being over home plate, between the tops of the knees and midway between the top of the shoulders and the top of the pants (see Figure 2.4).

FIGURE 2.4
The strike zone.

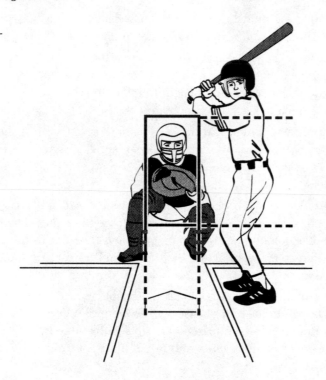

A few general pitching rules to impart to your players include

■ After a pitcher begins her motion toward home plate, she must complete it. Otherwise, a *balk* is called and all baserunners advance one base.

■ A pitcher cannot intentionally throw at a hitter.

■ A pitcher can't spit on the ball or rub any foreign substance on it.

Hitting Rules

Players must hit in the batting order you create. It's an automatic out if a player hits out of turn.

Many leagues allow designated hitters, meaning 9 players are in the field but a 10th player is in the batting order. This player takes his regular turn at bat but doesn't play in the field. (Of course, the player can be subbed in, just as any player can be.)

A batter must stand with both feet in the batter's box (see Figure 2.5). The lines of the box are considered part of the box; the feet can be on the lines but not outside them. After the pitcher begins her windup, the batter can't step out of the box.

FIGURE 2.5

The batter must stand in the bat-ter's box.

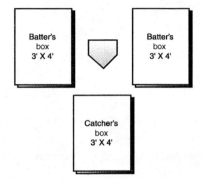

If a batter hits a ball with one or both feet on the ground outside the box, the batter is automatically out, whether the ball goes fair or foul. For other ways batters can make outs, see the following sidebar, "You're Out!"

"YOU'RE OUT!"

A batter is out when any of the following occurs:

- She is called out on strikes or swings and misses at strike three and the ball is caught by the catcher. Also, a batter is out if she tips a foul into the catcher's mitt on the third strike. (If the ball isn't caught and there are less than two outs with a runner on first, the batter is out. If there are two outs and a runner is on first and the ball isn't caught by the catcher, the batter must be tagged out by the catcher or thrown out at first base.)

- She bunts foul on the third strike.

- She hits a ball in the air that is caught by a fielder before it hits the ground.

- She hits a fair ball on the ground and the ball is in a defensive player's possession, with the player touching first base, before the batter/runner arrives at first.

- She runs outside the base path, interfering with the fielding of the ball or with the throw to first.

- She interferes with the catcher fielding or throwing the ball.

- Her own fair ball touches her before a fielder touches it. For this to happen, the batter has to be out of the batter's box.

- She hits a pop-up to the infield and the umpire calls the infield fly rule.

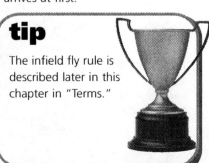

tip

The infield fly rule is described later in this chapter in "Terms."

Fielding Rules

The main fielding rules your players need to know include

▓ Force plays

▓ Tag plays

▓ The infield fly rule

▓ Defensive and offensive interference

Force Play

When a runner is forced to attempt to advance to the next base on a ground ball, it's called a *force play*. This happens when all preceding bases are occupied. Thus, the four situations in which one or more runners are forced to advance are as follows:

▓ Runner on first base

▓ Runners on first and second base

▓ Runners on first, second, and third base

▓ Runners on first and third base (only the runner on first is forced to advance; see Figure 2.6)

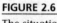
FIGURE 2.6
The situations in which runners are forced to advance on a ground ball. When runners are on first and third, only the runner on first is forced to advance.

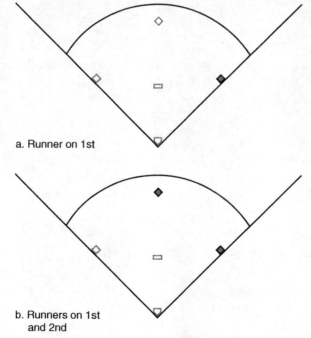

a. Runner on 1st

b. Runners on 1st and 2nd

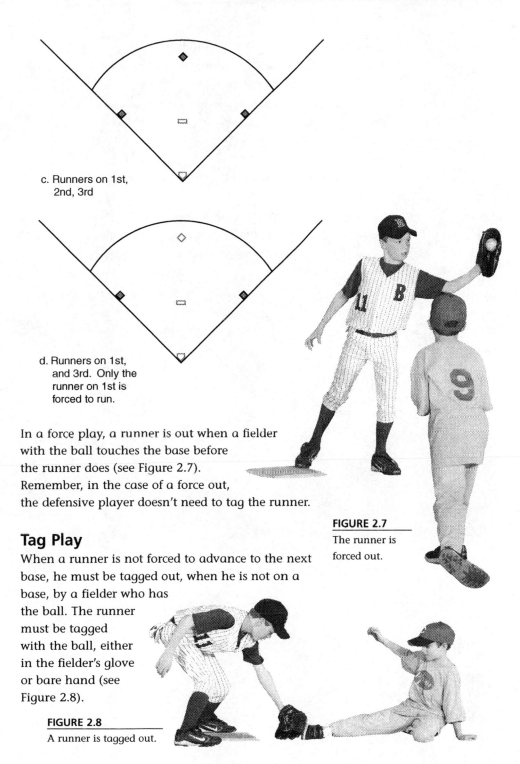

c. Runners on 1st,
   2nd, 3rd

d. Runners on 1st,
   and 3rd. Only the
   runner on 1st is
   forced to run.

In a force play, a runner is out when a fielder
with the ball touches the base before
the runner does (see Figure 2.7).
Remember, in the case of a force out,
the defensive player doesn't need to tag the runner.

Tag Play

When a runner is not forced to advance to the next
base, he must be tagged out, when he is not on a
base, by a fielder who has
the ball. The runner
must be tagged
with the ball, either
in the fielder's glove
or bare hand (see
Figure 2.8).

FIGURE 2.7
The runner is
forced out.

FIGURE 2.8
A runner is tagged out.

Runners must be tagged out in these situations:

■ Runner on second. With no runner on first forcing him to run when a ball is hit, a runner on second must be tagged out.

■ Runner on third. Similar to the situation of a runner on second base, when a runner is on third and runners are not on first and second as well, the runner on third is not forced to run and must be tagged out if she decides to leave the base.

■ Runners on second and third (neither runner is forced to advance and must be tagged to be put out).

■ Runners on first and third (the runner on first is forced to advance, but the runner on third is not and must be tagged to be put out; see Figure 2.9).

FIGURE 2.9

The situations in which runners must be tagged to be put out.

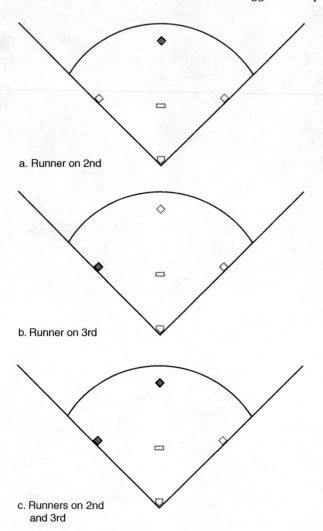

a. Runner on 2nd

b. Runner on 3rd

c. Runners on 2nd and 3rd

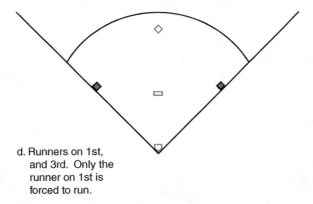

d. Runners on 1st,
and 3rd. Only the
runner on 1st is
forced to run.

Infield Fly Rule

This rule is in effect to stop a fielder from intentionally dropping an infield pop-up to trick any runners on base (thus perhaps getting a double play as opposed to recording a single out). The infield fly rule must be called by the umpire as the ball is in the air. The umpire should call this rule for any fair fly ball that can be caught in the infield with normal effort. It can only be called in these situations:

- With runners on first and second and fewer than two outs
- With the bases loaded and fewer than two outs

After the umpire calls an infield fly rule, the batter is automatically out and runners can stay at their bases or attempt to advance at their own risk.

Defensive Interference

This occurs when a defensive player who is not making a play on the ball impedes the progress of a baserunner. When this happens, the umpire calls the ball dead and the runner is allowed to advance to the next base, or to the base that the umpire believes the runner would have advanced to, had he not been impeded.

Offensive Interference

A baserunner can be called out for offensive interference if he interferes with a fielder trying to field the ball. Offensive interference can be called whether the interference was intentional or not.

Baserunning Rules

There are many baserunning rules. Here we'll consider the basics for these rules:

- Leadoffs and steals
- Ground ball situations

- Tagging up on fly balls
- Running beyond first base
- Runner being hit by a batted ball
- Running out of the baseline
- Making outs on the base paths

Leadoffs and Steals

Generally at the younger levels, leadoffs and steals are not allowed. Sometimes, however, by age 9 or 10, leadoffs and steals are allowed. Check with your league on this.

The main considerations here are these: Are leadoffs allowed? If leadoffs are not allowed, at what point can the runner leave the base? Sometimes the runner is allowed to leave as soon as the pitcher pitches; sometimes the runner can't leave the base until the ball is hit or is caught by (or gets by) the catcher.

Sometimes leadoffs might be allowed, but steals might not be. Finally, leadoffs and steals might be permitted. Find out what your league allows and coach your players appropriately.

Ground Ball Situations

Your baserunners need to know what to do when a ground ball is hit. You've just learned about ground-ball situations that force baserunners to advance to the next base and about ground balls that do not force them to advance. Just as your fielders need to know what to do in these situations, your baserunners need to know as well.

Coaches at first and third base should inform their baserunners of the situation, letting them know when they have to run and when they don't.

Tagging Up on Fly Balls

When a fly ball is caught with less than two outs, the runner must tag up (touch her base) after the catch is made before attempting to advance to the next base. If the runner leaves her base too early, the defense can appeal to the umpire before the next pitch and a fielder can step on the base with the ball in his possession. If the umpire agrees that the runner left the base early, the runner is called out. The umpire won't call the runner out unless the defense appeals the play in this way before the next pitch, however.

Running Beyond First Base

Another important rule to pass on is the rule that allows batter/runners to run beyond first base after touching the bag, so long as they don't turn toward second.

(If they turn toward second, they run the risk of being tagged out while being off the base. Coach your runners to run past the bag and turn to the right, toward foul territory, before returning to first base.) Many younger players think they have to stop directly on the bag, and slow down as they near first base to do so. Instruct them to run hard *through* first base, not slowing until they have touched the bag.

Runner Being Hit by a Batted Ball

If a fairly batted ball hits a runner before a fielder touches the ball, the runner is out, unless he is on base.

Running Out of the Baseline

A runner cannot run out of the baseline unless he is doing so to avoid contact with a fielder trying to field the ball. Otherwise, the runner is called out for running out of the baseline, which stretches three feet on either side of the direct line between the bases (see Figure 2.10).

FIGURE 2.10

The baseline extends three feet on either side of the direct line between the bases.

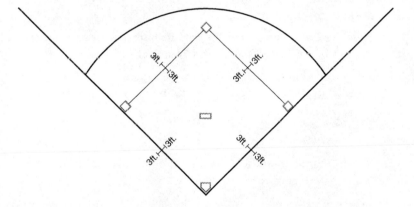

Making Outs on the Base Paths

You've read about runners who have been put out by being forced out at a base, tagged out between bases, called out on an appeal play for leaving base too early on a caught fly ball, called out for interfering with a defensive player who is trying to field the ball, and called out for running out of the baseline. A few other ways a runner can be put out include

- Being on the same base as another runner (one of the runners must be tagged out for the out to occur)
- Passing a runner who had been ahead of him on the base paths
- Missing a base and advancing to the next base (the play must be appealed by a fielder who holds the ball while she touches the missed base before the next pitch; the umpire will not automatically call the runner out).

How the Game Is Played

You've been introduced to the basics of the game, in terms of pitching, hitting, fielding, and baserunning rules. Here you learn the rudiments of how the game is played—that is, the general parameters that guide it from inning to inning.

The visiting team bats first in a game; the home team bats last. A team bats until three outs are recorded. (Some leagues also have a maximum-runs-per-half-inning rule; for example, a team can't score more than five runs in an inning, even if it hasn't made three outs.)

Batters try to get on base any way they can—by a hit, a walk, an error—and attempt to score by advancing safely around the bases. A run is scored if a runner advances legally and safely to first, second, and third and then touches home plate before three outs are made.

Fielders try to get the batters and runners out—by strikeout, ground out, fly out, tag out, or any other way that batters and runners can make an out.

Batters follow the batting order the coach makes, although coaches can substitute as their league rules allow.

If the home team is ahead after the visitors have had their final at-bat, the home team doesn't bat in the bottom of the final inning.

If the game is tied at the end of regulation, it goes into extra innings until a winner is determined, unless the league has rules that state otherwise.

Terms

The following terms should help you become familiar with the language, rules, and situations you will encounter as you coach your team:

- **Balk**—A balk occurs when a pitcher stops his motion toward home plate or makes another illegal move after beginning to pitch. Runners advance one base.

- **Ball**—A ball is called on any pitch that is out of the strike zone and not swung at by the batter.

- **Bunt**—Either to move baserunners up or to deceive the defense, a batter bunts at the ball rather than swinging at it. The batter tries to let the bat "catch" the ball, lightly tapping it a short way into the infield, generally down the first or third base line.

- **Choke up**—A batter chokes up on the bat when she moves her hands up the bat handle. This is done to gain greater bat control.

- **Count**—The count refers to balls and strikes. A 3-and-2 count means three balls and two strikes on the batter. The ball count is always given before the strike count.

- **Defensive interference**—As noted earlier, this occurs when a defensive player who is not making a play on the ball impedes the progress of a baserunner.

- **Designated hitter**—When rules allow, a 10th hitter can be inserted anywhere in the batting order. This hitter takes his regular turn at bat but does not play in the field.

- **Double**—This is a two-base hit; the batter ends up on second base without benefit of an error.

- **Double play**—This occurs when the defense records two outs on a single batted ball.

- **Dropped third strike**—When the catcher drops the third strike and no runner is on first base (or if a runner is on first with two out), the batter/runner must be put out by either being tagged with the ball or being thrown out at first base. This rule is often modified at lower levels of play.

- **Error**—When a fielder misplays a ball that allows a batter to reach base or a baserunner to advance, the fielder is charged with an error.

- **Fielder's choice**—This occurs when a fielder allows a batter to reach first base safely as the fielder attempts to put out a baserunner at another base.

- **Force play**—When a runner is forced to attempt to advance to the next base on a ground ball, it's called a force play. This happens when all preceding bases are occupied.

- **Foul ball**—A foul ball is any ball hit into foul territory. Note that when a ball touches ground in fair territory and then rolls foul after it has passed first or third base, it is a fair ball.

- **Foul tip**—A foul tip occurs when the batter tips the ball with her bat. With two strikes, a foul tip must be caught by the catcher for a strikeout to be recorded; if a two-strike foul tip is dropped, the batter is not out.

- **Hit by pitch**—When the batter is hit by a pitch, he is awarded first base, unless the umpire judges that the batter could have gotten out of the way of the pitch but intentionally remained in the way. (When a bat is swung, the hands are considered part of the bat. If, on a swing, the pitch hits a hand, the batter is not considered to have been hit by the pitch. If, however, the batter *doesn't* swing at the ball and is hit on a hand, that *is* considered being hit by the pitch.)

- **Home run**—This occurs when a batter hits the ball in fair territory over the fence. An inside-the-park home run occurs on a hit in which the batter is able to make it home without being thrown out (and with no errors being made).

- **Infield fly rule**—This rule, as explained earlier, should be called by the umpire for any fair fly ball that can be caught in the infield with normal effort. It can only be called with runners on first and second or with the bases loaded and fewer than two outs. The batter is automatically out.

- **Inning**—An inning is made up of three outs for each team, with the visiting team batting in the top half of the inning and the home team batting in the bottom half.

- **Leadoff**—In some leagues, a runner can lead off his base (that is, move off the base he's occupying and take some steps toward the next base). Many leagues for younger players prohibit leadoffs. Be aware that the runner can be tagged out while taking a leadoff. A pitcher or catcher can attempt a *pick-off* by throwing to the defensive player at the base where the runner is so the defensive player can tag the runner out. Coach your runners to come back to the base after each pitch that is not hit before attempting another leadoff.

- **Offensive interference**—A baserunner can be called out for offensive interference if she interferes with a fielder trying to field the ball.

- **Run batted in**—A player is awarded a run batted in (RBI) when his hit scores a runner (including himself on a home run). An RBI is also awarded when a runner scores on a sacrifice fly or a groundout (except in the case of a double play; no RBI is awarded here even if a run scores). No RBI is awarded if a runner scores on a wild pitch, a passed ball, or an error. Batters can get more than one RBI on one hit.

- **Running out of the baseline**—As described earlier, a baserunner is called out for running out of the baseline, unless he is doing so to avoid interfering with a fielder fielding a ball.

- **Sacrifice bunt**—When a batter successfully bunts with the intent of moving one or more runners up a base, that batter is awarded a sacrifice and is not charged with an official time at bat.

- **Sacrifice fly**—When a baserunner scores after tagging up and advancing on a fly out, the batter is credited with a sacrifice fly and an RBI. He is not charged with an official time at bat.

■ **Scoring position**—Runners are considered to be in scoring position when they are on either second or third base.

■ **Single**—A batter hits a single when she is credited with a base hit and ends up on first base.

■ **Squeeze play**—A squeeze play is a bunt with a runner on third base. A *safety squeeze* means the runner on third breaks for home only after the batter has made contact with the ball; a *suicide squeeze* means the runner breaks for home as soon as the rules allow, and before the batter has a chance to make contact.

■ **Steal**—Some leagues allow baserunners to try to steal bases—that is, to take off for the next base as the pitcher is preparing to pitch or is in the midst of pitching.

■ **Strike**—A strike is any pitch in the strike zone that is not swung at or a pitch that is swung at and missed or hit foul. If a bunter offers at a pitch and misses it, it's a strike. The only time a batter can strike out when the third strike is a foul ball is if the foul comes on a bunt attempt.

■ **Tag play**—When a runner is not forced to advance to the next base, he must be tagged out by a fielder who has the ball when the runner is not on a base.

■ **Tag up**—A baserunner must tag her base after a fly ball is caught before attempting to advance to the next base.

■ **Triple**—This is a hit in which the batter safely makes it to third base with no errors occurring.

■ **Triple play**—This occurs when the defense records three outs on one batted ball.

■ **Walk**—A walk is a base on balls, in which the batter is awarded first base after taking (not swinging at) four balls out of the strike zone.

Signals

Signals are part of all sports. There are two types of signals in baseball:

■ Umpire signals

■ Coach signals

Let's first take a look at umpire signals.

Umpire Signals

There are relatively few signals umpires need to make, but you need to know them, as do your players. Figures 2.11–2.16 show some of the most common umpire signals.

note

Many volunteer umpires aren't used to signaling and haven't been trained to use signals. If you're unclear of a call, find a reasonable way to ask the umpire to clarify his call.

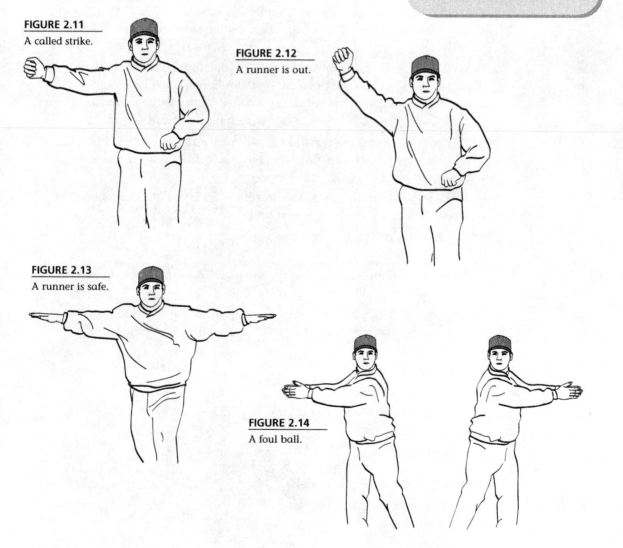

FIGURE 2.11
A called strike.

FIGURE 2.12
A runner is out.

FIGURE 2.13
A runner is safe.

FIGURE 2.14
A foul ball.

FIGURE 2.15
A fair ball.

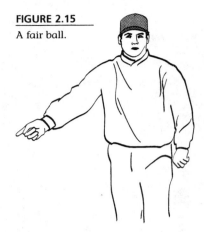

FIGURE 2.16
Time out.

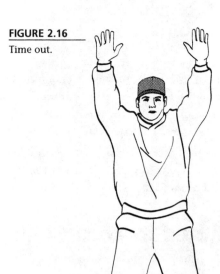

Coach Signals

You might use signals for your batters; the third base coach normally delivers these signals. If you do use signals, keep them simple and easy to remember. You might devise signals for swing away, take (don't swing), bunt, hit-and-run, and steal. Whatever your signals, make sure your players know them.

You might see Major League or college coaches giving a complex set of signals. The complexity they use can be very confusing for your players' age level. Keep to simple signs.

For example, for a bunt, you could tell your players that when you touch the bill of your cap, they should bunt on the next pitch. If you touch an elbow, that signifies you want your runners to steal. When you swipe your hand across your chest, this might tell your hitters to take the next pitch. These are simple signs, as you can see, and such signs are appropriate for the level of player you are working with.

caution

The other team might figure out that, if you touch the bill of your cap, the batter will be bunting. This takes the surprise out of your bunt attempt and makes the play easier for the defense. If you suspect that the other team has figured out your signals, switch your signs. Tell your players why you are doing this, and keep the new signs simple, too. Stealing signs is typically considered poor sportsmanship at lower levels of baseball, but it does happen and you should be prepared to handle the situation if it happens to you.

Keep on Learning

Knowing the rules is one of your primary duties because it influences how you coach and instruct your players and which strategies you might use during a game. So, know the rules, impart them to your players, and coach accordingly.

You can find more in-depth information on baseball rules on various websites and from youth baseball organizations.

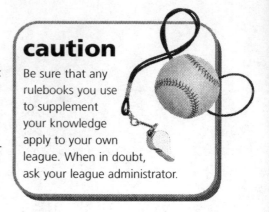

caution

Be sure that any rulebooks you use to supplement your knowledge apply to your own league. When in doubt, ask your league administrator.

Teaching Rules to Your Players

To help your players know the rules, you need to know three things, in this order:

1. What your players *need* to know

2. What they *do* know

3. How to best impart what your players need to learn

Your players need to know the basics: the number of innings, the number of outs per inning, the strike zone, what constitutes an out, the basics of baserunning, batting, pitching, and fielding rules.

Some of that—for example, the number of innings, the number of outs per inning, and similar information—should be easy for players to remember. Some of the other rules will likely take more time for them to learn and understand—for example, when it's a force play, when it's a tag play, what defensive and offensive interference are, and so on.

As you begin practicing and place your kids in game situations in practice, it will become evident which rules they know and which rules they don't know. At that point, it's up to you to make sure they learn what they need.

How should you go about teaching the rules to your players? Doing your best imitation of a classroom lecturer is definitely *not* the way to go. That will hold your players' attention for less than the time it takes to run from home to first base.

There are some effective ways you can teach the rules, though. Here are four ways you can help your players learn the rules of baseball:

- Situational plays
- Practice games
- Brief discussions
- Players' experiences

Let's take a look at each way.

Situational Plays

If you want your players to learn about force plays, set up some plays to help them learn. With players at each infield position and using baserunners, test your players' understanding of how they should respond in various situations.

For example, put a baserunner on first base and tell the infield there is one out and they should make whatever play is appropriate. Then hit a ground ball to, say, the shortstop. Does the shortstop field the grounder and force the runner at second base? Does the second baseman break to second and prepare to take the throw from the shortstop? If so, they get it. If not, explain what they should be doing: going for the force out at second and trying to complete the double play by also forcing the batter/runner out at first base, if possible.

Then place a runner at second (no runner at first). Hit a ground ball to the third baseman near the bag. Does he attempt to field the ball and step on third base, thinking he's forcing out the runner? Or does he hold the runner at second and throw the batter/runner out at first base?

Place runners in various positions, hit the ball to various infielders, and coach your players according to what you see they need to learn.

You can use situational plays to teach anything: force plays, tag plays, tagging up, making relay throws from the outfield, making throws to every base, and so on. And you can use the plays to instruct baserunners, too, even if the focus is on the defense. The main point is to plan how to use your practice time and base your activities on what kids need to learn and improve on.

Practice Games

You can also use short practice games—maybe playing a few innings—to see how much your players know and how they respond to various situations, and to teach them the correct response when they're unclear on what they should do. In this setting, your teaching focus is broader; you provide instruction in whatever area you see your players need it. In one moment, it might be on baserunning tactics; the next moment it might be on hitting the cutoff man on a hit to the outfield; a few minutes later, you might find the opportunity to clarify when to make a tag and how to make it.

When you use practice games in this manner, you have a couple of choices: You can briefly stop play and instruct your players as the need arises, or you can note what you need to tell them and then discuss your point(s) at the end of practice. In general, it's best to briefly stop the play and get your teaching point across without belaboring your point and then let play resume. The best teaching moment is, after all, on the spot. Just get in, get out, and let the flow continue. In baseball you can do this easily with the brief breaks between each play.

Brief Discussions

The end-of-practice discussion is also a good time to briefly teach or remind players of a rule (or anything else important) that they appeared to have difficulty understanding in that practice.

For example, you might say, "I noticed that sometimes we're forgetting to tag up on fly balls. What does it mean to tag up?" Ideally, at least a few players will know what it means. If a player offers a correct answer, repeat it for everyone to hear. If no one responds correctly, tell them what tagging up means and make a note to work on that situation during the next practice.

Use these practice-ending discussions to briefly make a point, ideally a point that ties in directly to the activities of that practice. Don't drone on about various rules, especially if they don't relate to what the kids experienced that day. Kids learn better when the learning is practical and in context with what they're doing.

> **tip**
>
> When you offer praise for correct answers, this encourages players to respond to future questions. Of course, never belittle players for incorrect answers. It makes your players feel bad, and they will be less likely to participate in other team discussions.

> **note**
>
> In the next chapter you'll learn effective ways to communicate to your players, both during practice and in end-of-practice discussions.

Players' Experiences

Imagine the coach that teaches his players the rules by the book. He sits them down in orderly rows, lectures them for 50 minutes, and then gives them a written test, which they all ace. (I told you you'd have to use your imagination.)

Then the first game arrives, and the players have no idea when a force play is in order, or a tag play, or what offensive and defensive interference are. As far as they know, the infield fly rule must have something to do with pest control.

Book knowledge can't take the place of firsthand experience. Players learn the rules best when they see them applied in the practices and games they play in, especially when they are involved in the plays. *Then* the rules begin to register.

And that's good news because it means you don't have to spend your time lecturing to them about all the rules; you have to instruct along the way, as they play. And everyone—yourself included—has more fun that way.

Part of your job as coach is to reinforce your players' learning from practice to practice and game to game. As you observe their performances and discover what they need to learn, you can teach them not only the skills of baseball, but also the rules.

THE ABSOLUTE MINIMUM

This chapter focused on the basic rules of baseball—the general structure of the game as well as specific rules for pitching, hitting, fielding, and baserunning. In addition, it provided terms you need to know, umpiring signals, coaches' signals, and ways to help your players learn. Points to keep in mind include

■ You need to know not only the basic rules of baseball, but also any specific modifications your league has in place.

■ Your players need to know the basic rules, and part of your responsibility is to determine what they do know and what they need to learn.

■ After you know what your players need to learn, plan for effective ways to teach them the rules. These ways include using situational plays in practice, using practice games as teaching tools, holding brief end-of-practice discussions, and reinforcing players' learning through their own experiences gained through practices and games.

■ You can expand your own knowledge of the rules by finding resources through your own league, through youth baseball organizations, and through resources you can find in your library or on the Web.

Your players need to know the rules to compete in games, but coaches often don't teach rules because they're so focused on teaching skills. You'll be a step ahead if you take the time to also teach your players the rules they need to know.

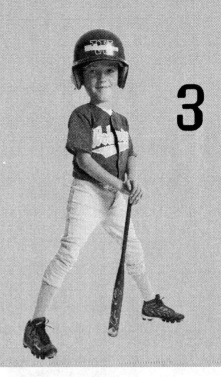

3

COMMUNiCATiON KEYS

As a coach, you're called on to do a lot of communicating. You address players, parents, other coaches, league administrators, and umpires. You communicate in person, on the phone, in writing, one on one, and within group settings. How well you communicate with these groups significantly influences how successful your season is, how enjoyable it is, and how much your players learn.

Of course, you've been communicating all your life. It can't be that hard, right?

Right and wrong. If you haven't coached or taught before, and if you aren't used to instructing and leading youngsters, then you are entering uncharted territory.

Consider this chapter your roadmap to help you chart that territory.

The 10 keys, presented first, will help you hone your communication skills as a coach. These keys are written with players in mind, but they apply to all groups you will communicate with. Following the keys, we'll focus on the specifics of communicating with parents, league administrators, opponents, and umpires.

10 Keys to Being a Good Communicator

Most people tend to think only of the verbal side of communication. That's important, but there's so much more to being a good communicator. Here are 10 keys to good communication:

1. Know your message.
2. Make sure you are understood.
3. Deliver your message in the proper context.
4. Use appropriate emotions and tones.
5. Adopt a healthy communication style.
6. Be receptive.
7. Provide helpful feedback.
8. Be a good nonverbal communicator.
9. Be consistent.
10. Be positive.

Know Your Message

Coach Caravelli gathers his players at the practice field and says, "Alright, guys, today we're going to learn how to bunt." With a bat in his hands, he stands in the batter's box and mimics a bunter. "What you want to do is wait for the pitch to come to you and then push your bat toward the ball, like this." He makes an exaggerated pushing motion with the bat.

"But Coach, my dad says you're just supposed to let the ball meet the bat, almost like you're trying to catch it with the bat," one player says.

Coach Caravelli considers this a moment before saying, "Actually, let's just focus on swinging away today. You guys like to hit, right? Who wants to bunt, anyway?"

The player was right; Coach Caravelli didn't know the technique for bunting. He didn't really know his message.

Three issues are involved in knowing your message. You need to

- Know the skills and rules you need to teach.
- Read situations and respond appropriately.
- Provide accurate and clear information.

Know the Skills and Rules

Coach Caravelli didn't know how to teach the skill of bunting. He might be a smooth, coherent, and clear speaker, but that's not going to help his players learn how to bunt. Smoothness doesn't make up for lack of knowledge. You have to know the skills and rules.

Read the Situation

As Coach Caravelli teaches his players how to correctly execute a rundown situation on the base paths, Kenny and Sam are quietly goofing off, not paying attention. But Coach Caravelli doesn't address the situation because they're not really disrupting his instruction and he's a little behind schedule. As his players begin to practice rundowns, Kenny and Sam are not executing as instructed. They are not running the runner back to the previous base, and they are making too many throws.

So, Coach Caravelli stops the action and tells them how to properly execute a rundown. Then he lets them proceed.

Coach Caravelli delivered an important part of the message—Kenny and Sam need to know how to execute a rundown—but that was only part of the message he should have delivered. The real issue here was that the players weren't paying attention, and Coach Caravelli didn't correct that situation when it was occurring.

He should have corrected that on the spot. Barring that, he should have told Kenny and Sam that the reason they didn't know how to execute a rundown was because they weren't listening when he was teaching how to do so, and that they need to listen to his instruction the first time around.

Sometimes knowing your message goes beyond understanding the content. You have to read the situation as well and tailor your message accordingly.

warning

Eloquently stating and aptly showing how to perform a skill doesn't mean you're a good communicator if you can't keep your players' attention.

Provide Accurate and Clear Information

Knowing the content of your message isn't enough. You need to be able to deliver that content clearly and accurately.

Imagine a portion of a coach's preseason letter to parents reading like this:

> *"I'm really looking forward to coaching your child this season. Our first practice is next Monday at 6 p.m. Please make sure your child remembers to bring a glove!"*

Too bad the coach didn't remember to note *where* the first practice is being held. As a result of not being clear in his letter, he'll have to spend a lot of time on the phone calling parents to deliver the information.

The same goes for teaching skills. Perhaps you know the proper technique for swinging a bat, but your instruction is so technical and confusing that your players are worse off than if they'd received no instruction at all! They're confused, you're frustrated, and no one learns how to hit.

Know what information you need to deliver, and deliver it clearly so that all concerned understand. That's sometimes easier said than done.

Make Sure You Are Understood

As you can imagine, if you are not clear with your directives, you can create a lot of confusion. Take the following example:

> "Okay, Dion," Coach Hagan says, "the next time on a throw like that from the outfield, take a crow hop to give you a little momentum and power. All right? Let's try it again."

Dion gives Coach Hagan a puzzled look, but Coach Hagan, in the midst of conducting a fielding drill, doesn't notice. He's already preparing to hit the ball again. Dion just hopes it's not to him because he has no idea what a "crow hop" is.

Just because something is clear to you doesn't mean it is clear to whomever you're delivering your message to, be it a player, a parent, an administrator, or anyone else. You need to watch for understanding and be ready to clarify your message if the person on the receiving end is confused.

When you state your message clearly and simply, you increase your chances of being understood. But don't count on that; instead, watch your players' facial expressions and read their body language. If they look confused or unsure of what to do, state your instruction again, making sure you use language they understand.

And watch how you say things: When you encourage a runner to "take an extra base," he might not understand that you mean to advance to the next base. Likewise, "hit the cutoff man" doesn't help your right fielder if he doesn't know what a cutoff man is.

Speak in language your players understand, and watch for their understanding.

Deliver Your Message in the Proper Context

Karim, playing second base in the first game of the season, has just botched what Coach Grantham felt was a perfect double-play ball. Though he had time to get in front of the ball, he tried to backhand it and began his flip to the shortstop before he had control of the ball. No outs were recorded.

tip

A quizzical eye, a slumping shoulder, or a glazed look on a player's face speaks volumes. When you are able to understand your players' nonverbal communication, you are on the road to being a better communicator yourself.

Coach Grantham takes a few steps out of the dugout and cups his hands to his mouth. "Hey, Karim! Get in front of the ball! Get down on it and watch it into your glove, like this!" Coach Grantham models the proper technique to field a ground ball. "Then make the snap throw, like this!" He makes a phantom toss to a make-believe shortstop.

What's wrong with this? First, it's probably humiliating for Karim to have everyone in the park witness his coach trying to instruct him on how to field a ground ball. Second, it's not the time or place to give detailed instruction—that should be done in practice, not in games. The instruction itself wasn't incorrect; the timing of it was.

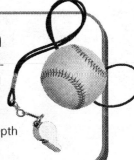

caution

Players' focus during games should be on the game itself, not on you giving them in-depth instruction.

So, consider your context for delivering your message. Give brief reminders of tactical or skill execution during games, but save the teaching for practices.

Use Appropriate Emotions and Tones

Emotions are a natural part of baseball. Both you and your players (and their parents) can expect to experience a range of emotions throughout the season. In terms of communicating with others, your emotions can significantly affect your message.

How? Let's look at a few examples:

Situation: The opposing team has a runner on third with one out. The batter lofts a fly ball to medium center field. Janet, your center fielder, camps under the ball but drops it in her haste to make a quick throw to the plate. The runner scores and the batter is safe at first base.

Response #1: "Come on, Janet! That was a can of corn! You should have had that easily!"

Response #2: "That's okay, guys! Let's get this next out, now. Infield, there's a force at second."

Don't ever berate a player, publicly or privately. Remember that even major league players make plenty of errors. Your players are going to make errors; what they need is instruction, if they're not sure how to make a play, and encouragement regardless. Help them to keep their focus on the game, not on how well they're pleasing you.

Situation: You are moments away from beginning the game that will decide your league championship.

Response #1: "All right, this is it, guys! There's no tomorrow. We've been playing to get to this game all year long. Show them what you're made of. I want to feel that championship trophy in my hands at the end of the game. How about you? Are you ready to go out and win?"

Response #2: "Okay, let's play baseball like we know how. Keep your focus on the fundamentals. Take good cuts, don't swing at bad pitches, and watch that ball into your glove before you try to throw it. Let's go out and have some fun, all right?"

Pep talks are better saved for the movies. Such talks often backfire because they get kids so sky high that they can't perform well. Your players need to focus on playing sound, fundamental baseball. Remind them of that and tell them to have fun:

Situation: In batting practice, Terrell keeps bailing out (stepping with his front foot toward third base).

Response #1: "Hey, Terrell, you look like you're ready to run to third base, not first base, the way you're stepping out! You're halfway into the dugout with your right foot!"

Response #2: "Step toward the pitcher, Terrell. Keep your front foot in there. You can do it."

Sarcasm will get you nowhere. Terrell doesn't need sarcasm, or any type of humor. He needs instruction and encouragement.

Adopt a Healthy Communication Style

A lot of what you've been reading has to do with your communication style— whether you over-coach during games, offering too much instruction; whether you keep your emotions in check, or are too excitable or high-strung; what your tone is as you communicate; and so on. But there is more to consider concerning your communication style. It has to do with the bigger picture, with how you communicate on a daily basis. It has more to do with personality, outlook, and attitude than with reacting to a specific moment. And some styles are more effective than others.

Here are a few of the less-effective styles some coaches fall into:

- **Always talking, never listening**—Some coaches feel if they're not constantly talking, they're not providing the proper instruction their players need. Carried to the extreme, some feel that their players have nothing to say. Coaches who always talk and never listen tend to have players who stand around more in practice because their coach is talking, and those coaches don't get to know their players, thus missing out on one of the real joys of coaching baseball. *Deliver the messages you need to deliver, but don't feel you have to be talking throughout the entire practice.*

- **Always in control, too directive**—Some coaches run practices like drill sergeants, snapping orders at players, exerting their authority, and squelching fun wherever it begins to appear. When practice doesn't go exactly as they have choreographed it, they become irked. When players don't progress according to schedule, it drives them crazy. So do rainouts. *Be in control of practice, yes, but don't squelch the fun and don't obsess over things you can't control.*

- **Not in control, too passive**—Other coaches take the opposite tack, either because they're unsure of themselves or they're too laid-back and give the impression that *no* one is in charge. They don't provide the guidance or discipline players need. Not comfortable in the spotlight, they avoid it, and discipline problems begin to crop up. *If you're a quiet or laid-back person, don't change your personality but do exert your authority as coach. You can be in charge and provide instruction without being loud and obnoxious.*

- **Seeking perfection**—There's a fine line between seeking to improve and seeking perfection. When coaches cross over the line into perfectionism, they are rarely satisfied with anything. Their fielders record the outs, but their technique is not quite right. Hitters get hits, but they have flaws in their swings. Even the fields are not manicured to these coaches' satisfaction. Players are on edge when they play for a perfectionist coach; their focus turns from playing the game to pleasing the coach. *Help your players improve their skills, but allow them margin for error. You can strive for improvement without putting added stress on the kids. Celebrate improvement even if it's still not picture-perfect.*

- **Not in control of emotions**—Some coaches throw up their hands in frustration when players are trying hard but having difficulty learning a skill. They shout in anger at a questionable call made by a volunteer umpire. Their voices drip with sarcasm when players ask them something they feel the players should know. They respond with overzealous enthusiasm when their team scores a run in a tight game, and this response is seen by all as unsporting behavior. *The point is not to suppress all your emotions, but to be in control of them. Consider the message you send with the emotion you show. Do suppress any urge to show your frustration toward kids who are trying to learn the skills, as well as any desire to express your anger on the field. Maintain your respect for the people involved in all situations. Your players need you to be steady and need to know what to expect from you.*

- **Not aware of nonverbal communication**—Some coaches watch what they say but not what they do. They express their frustration or anger nonverbally, and if someone confronts them about that expression, they likely will say, "What? I didn't say anything." *Remember that you're communicating every second, whether verbally or nonverbally. Keep your nonverbal communication in line with your verbal communication, and make sure that both are positive, instructive, and encouraging.*

- **Buddy-buddy with the players**—It's good to be friendly with players, but it's inappropriate to try to be their friend. Coaches who do this show a lack of maturity as they try to impress their players with how cool they are. *Have fun with your players, but maintain the coach-player relationship. You're there to help them become better ballplayers, not to become their pal.*

So, what *should* your communication style be?

You should provide the instruction your players need in a way that helps them improve their skills. To do this, you need good listening skills as well as good speaking skills, and you need to be encouraging and positive as you instruct and correct. Maintain respect for your players as you communicate with them. Be friendly and open with them, but don't try to become their friend. Create an enjoyable learning environment, maintain control over your emotions, and watch your nonverbal communication.

When you adopt this type of communication style, you're paving the way for your players to learn the game, improve their skills, and enjoy the season.

Be Receptive

A common mistake of new coaches is to assume that their sole role in communicating is to *talk*. Athletes are there to receive instruction, to be coached. Their focus should be on listening to you, on soaking in your instruction, on carrying out your commands.

There's plenty of truth in those statements, but they don't reflect the *whole* truth. Give your players room to speak, to ask questions, to voice opinions or concerns. In doing so, you can get to know them better and are better tuned in to their needs. Thus, you are more likely to pick up on issues and problems you need to deal with; see the following sidebar, "Dealing with Issues As They Arise."

caution

Communication is a two-way street. If you make it one-way, athletes will eventually tune you out because you tuned them out when they attempted to talk to you.

Work at not only sending messages, but receiving them as well. As you talk to players, if you notice that their eyes are wandering or their bodies are turned partially away from you, they're sending you a message ("We're not really listening"). If their shoulders are slumped, their heads are down, or they're dragging their feet, they're sending one or more messages ("I'm tired"; "I'm discouraged"; "I'm bored"). If they're giving you a blank stare or have a dazed look, they're telling you they are tuning you out or are confused.

DEALING WITH ISSUES AS THEY ARISE

You might come across some discipline issues and other concerns you need to address as the season progresses. Here are some pointers on how to handle those issues:

- Let players know at the first practice how you expect them to behave, and let them know what the consequences of misbehavior will be. Write this down as well and give it to players or send it directly to their parents. This list needn't and shouldn't be long; it should be simple and clear and framed in a positive manner.
- Rather than just laying down the law, consider involving your players in making team rules. Do this at the first practice. When they take part in making the rules and setting the consequences for breaking them, they might be more apt to stick to the rules. Giving players this type of responsibility promotes their emotional and social growth.
- When a player misbehaves, follow through as you had said you would.
- Don't tolerate razzing of teammates, taunting of opposing players, or other poor sporting behavior. Put a stop to such behavior, and follow through on any prescribed penalties.
- When a player needs extra help at practice in learning a skill, try to provide it on the spot, ideally using an assistant coach or a parent who volunteers to help. If the help can't be provided during that practice, other options might be to provide further instruction immediately following the practice or immediately preceding the next practice, in a one-on-one situation, if possible.
- When a player needs medical attention, provide the appropriate care immediately. You'll learn about this care in Chapter 4, "Safety Principles."

Provide Helpful Feedback

Tyler has been having trouble in the infield. He tends to rush things, wanting to throw the ball before he has control of it, and as a result he makes a lot of errors. After one such error, Tyler and his teammates return to the bench after the inning is over.

> "Tyler, you need to field those grounders and make good throws to first base," Coach Dixon says.

Is Coach Dixon telling Tyler something he doesn't already know? Hardly. Is he helping Tyler improve his fielding technique? No. His feedback isn't helpful at all; if anything, it just adds to the pressure Tyler undoubtedly already feels.

Coach Dixon should focus on giving specific, practical feedback that will help Tyler improve his fielding. You'll learn about this type of feedback in Chapter 6, "Player Development." For now, know that such feedback is one of your duties in communicating with your players, and when it's given properly it can reap great dividends in terms of player improvement.

Be a Good Nonverbal Communicator

Studies have shown that up to 70% of communication is accomplished nonverbally. You just read about the importance of reading nonverbal cues—watching facial expressions and body language. You also have to pay attention to the nonverbal cues you send:

> "Way to go, Alex!" Coach Dintiman says, clapping his hands and smiling.

> "Way to go, Alex!" Coach Garner says, arms crossed tightly across his chest and a scowl on his face.

The same words were used, but Coach Garner sent a vastly different message from Coach Dintiman's.

Nonverbal messages are being sent constantly—both with and without words. Consider your facial expressions during practices and games. Sometimes it's appropriate to show that you're frustrated—for example, when kids are goofing off. But when kids are exerting themselves on the field and not executing well, keep your frustration in check. Consider what messages your expressions and body language are sending, and make sure those messages are what you *want* to be sending.

Be Consistent

Your players need consistency from you in three ways. They need consistency

- In the messages you send
- In how you treat them
- In your temperament and style

Consistent Messages

If you hear different messages from the same person on the same topic, what happens? You begin not to trust that person. The same happens if one week your players hear you say, "As the pitcher releases the ball, take a step toward the pitcher as you get ready to swing," only to hear you follow that the next week with, "There's no need to take a step as the pitcher releases the ball. Just pick up your front foot, set it down where you picked it up, and swing." Confusing? You bet. If you do this often, the players will not know what to believe, no matter what you say. Be sure you send consistent messages.

caution

Remember, if your body language conflicts with your words, players will be just as confused as if you told them one thing one day, and the opposite thing the next. Keep your body language in line with the verbal messages you send.

Consistent Treatment

Make sure you treat all your players in a similar fashion. If Dana breaks a team rule one week, and you discipline her accordingly, and the next week Zach breaks the same rule, but you overlook it because he's one of your best players, what message does that send to your team? That it's okay to break the rules if you're good enough?

Likewise, if you spend more of your time with your average and good players, in hopes of turning them into good and great players, respectively, what does that say to the lesser-skilled players? That they don't matter because they can't throw or hit as well as their teammates?

All your players need your attention and guidance to improve. They need to adhere to the same team rules and be treated the same way if they break those rules. And they all need to know that they are equally valued by you, regardless of their playing ability.

Consistent Style

They also need to know what to expect from you. If you are patient and encouraging one practice and moody or volatile the next, the learning environment suffers (as do the players). We all have mood swings, and we're not robots. But do strive to be even-keeled and consistent in your approach from practice to practice, setting aside any personal issues that might affect your mood and your communication with your players on any given day.

Be Positive

Kids learn best in a positive environment. Give them sound instruction, consistent encouragement, and plenty of understanding. Note, however, that being positive doesn't mean letting kids run all over you, and it doesn't mean having a Pollyanna attitude where you falsely praise your second baseman for knocking the ball down when she should have easily fielded it and thrown out the batter. It means you instruct and guide your players as they learn and practice skills and give them the sincere encouragement and praise they need as they work to hone their abilities. You'll learn more about how to use praise in Chapter 6.

note

These 10 keys not only apply to how you communicate with your players, but also should guide your communication with parents, umpires, other coaches, and administrators.

Communicating with Parents

While most communication happens between coaches and players, important communication takes place between coaches and parents, too. In this section, we'll consider the various times and ways you should communicate with parents and learn how to handle challenging situations and involve parents in positive ways throughout the season.

Preseason Meeting or Letter

You'll need to contact parents before the season begins. You can communicate the following information at a parents' meeting or through a letter. If you hold a parents' meeting, it's still helpful to give parents a handout that covers the items you talk about, so they can have written information to refer to later. In your preseason meeting or letter, consider including the following items:

- **Introduction**—Tell parents who you are, what your coaching background is (if you have one), and how you got involved coaching the team. Make this brief, but know that parents appreciate knowing a bit about who will be coaching their sons and daughters.

- **Your coaching philosophy**—Let parents know your approach to coaching, including your philosophy in terms of providing instruction, giving all players equal playing time, and so on. Tell them, briefly, *why* this is your philosophy and how it benefits the kids.

■ **The inherent risks**—Baseball has some inherent risks you need to make parents aware of. You should also let them know you have a plan in place to respond to injuries, and find out from parents any medical conditions their children have, as well as how the parents can be contacted in case of an emergency. You'll learn more about this in Chapter 4.

■ **Basic expectations**—State your expectations of players and parents, in a positive fashion, and let parents know what they and their children can expect of you as a coach.

■ **The practice schedule**—Include the day, date, time, and place of the first practice, and note the rest of the practice schedule, if you know it at this time.

■ **The game schedule**—If you know the game schedule, include that as well. If not, let parents know when they can expect to receive the schedule.

■ **Other information**—If you have some special event planned or want to invite parents to volunteer to help in various ways, inform parents in your meeting or letter.

■ **Your contact information**—Let parents know how and when they can contact you.

For a sample preseason letter, see Appendix A, "Sample Letter to Parents."

Preseason Call

Even with a preseason letter or meeting, it's wise to call parents of players before the first practice to remind them of the time and place of that practice. Otherwise, you'll likely have players who don't show up for the first practice.

During the Season

After the season is underway, you'll have numerous opportunities to communicate with parents: as kids are being dropped off or picked up at practice, after games, and on the phone or through email at other times of the week. Here are some pointers on doing so:

■ If you have a few minutes immediately before or after practice, that's a good time to meet parents, get to know them a little bit, match faces with names, and enlist help if you need it. It's also a good time to let parents know what they can do to help their child. For example, you could suggest to Ramon's parents that if they had time, they could work with him at home on fielding ground balls to his left, or you could let Tara's parents know she could use some practice judging fly balls. Parents like to know what they can do to help their son or daughter.

- Ask parents to let you know when their child is not going to be at a game. Also let them know they can talk with you about any concerns they have about their child.

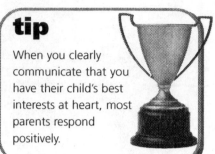

tip

When you clearly communicate that you have their child's best interests at heart, most parents respond positively.

- Let parents know what type of communication is allowed during games. Whatever boundaries you set here, do so with the players in mind and what will help them focus on the game the most. Some coaches prefer not to have any direct parental intervention during a game, meaning shouting encouragement from the stands is fine, but going to the bench to talk to their child is not. Other coaches don't mind parents coming by the bench and chatting briefly to the players; this is up to you. Just let parents know what your preferences are here, and ask that they respect them.

- Likewise, let parents know what's appropriate immediately after games. Many coaches like to spend 5 minutes or so talking to their players, reinforcing what went well and talking about what they still need to work on. At younger ages, post-game sometimes means snack time as well. Whatever your protocol, let parents know and let them know if and how they can be appropriately involved.

- Rainouts call for communicating with parents, too. If a game or practice is rained out, you can contact parents in whatever way you've set up: by yourself, with the aid of an assistant coach, or by phone tree (which you should have assigned beforehand).

Whichever way you decide, though, make sure parents are contacted by phone when a practice or game is rained out. Even if parents say email is a good way to contact them, chances are not all parents will check their email in time.

Be Understanding—and Set Boundaries

Most parents are there to cheer on their kids. Parents want to see their kids do their best, have fun, and succeed. It's thrilling for a parent to watch her child get a key hit, make a great play in the field, or slide home with the winning run. And it's painful for a parent to watch her son strike out or see her daughter make an error in a crucial situation. It's likely that parents experience more emotional highs and lows watching their children play than do the players and coaches who are directly involved in the game.

You need to understand the experience from the parents' point of view and create an environment that allows parents to be positively involved throughout the season. Indeed, you should encourage such participation. (For suggestions on how to do this, see the following sidebar "Involving Parents.")

At the same time, you need to set boundaries for parents and be prepared to handle situations that can detract from the players' experience. Some of those situations and boundaries are addressed in the following section, "Challenging Situations."

INVOLVING PARENTS

Some parents present challenges to coaches. But most want to support the team and its coach. Help parents know how they can be involved with your team in positive ways. Here are a few ideas:

- **Encourage support**—Ask parents to be positive and vocal in their support of each player and to display good sporting behavior. Their main role at games is to cheer on their team.

- **Ask for help**—If you don't have an assistant coach, ask if any parent would like to volunteer. Even if you do have an assistant, having parents volunteer to help at practice can be beneficial because you can break the players into smaller units and thus give them more swings, more fielding chances, and so on. Also, you might want to set up parents on a snack schedule, with a different parent or set of parents responsible for providing a team snack at each game. You also might set up a phone tree with parents so important information can be quickly passed on.

  In addition, if you and your assistant coach don't like to keep the scorebook, you might find that a parent wouldn't mind that task.

- **Build camaraderie**—Social gatherings are nice ways to build camaraderie among parents and team family members. Consider having a midseason potluck or pizza party to help families get to know each other better, or plan other social events that foster open communication and deepened relationships. And parents are often more than willing to step to the fore and organize such events—so let them!

Challenging Situations

You might not have any challenging situations with parents. But it's best to be prepared for those challenges and know how to respond, just in case. Following are some of the challenges coaches can face and suggestions for how to handle them.

Parents Who Coach from the Stands

At some time during the season, you might experience the following:

> "Bring the infield in! Cut off the run at the plate," one parent yells at one point in the game. "Come on, send in a pinch hitter," another yells in the next inning. "Lay down a bunt, Jason," a third parent shouts a little later.

It's one thing to encourage players from the stands; it's quite another to coach them from that vantage point. It's not a matter of whether the instruction is good; it's a matter of where that instruction is coming from. Coaching advice is your domain.

If you hear parents of your players coaching from the stands, remind your players to focus on what you say, not on what they hear elsewhere. Then, after the game, talk to the parents who were coaching from the stands. Tell them they need to focus their support on cheering on the team, not on telling them how to play. It's confusing and disconcerting for players to hear instruction from the stands, even if it's in line with what you've told them. And quite often that instruction flies in the face of what you've told them.

In any case, coaching from the stands is disruptive and inappropriate. Tell the offending parents this and request that they refrain from it in the future.

Parents Who Demand That You Coach Their Child Differently

There is also the possibility you will have parents who just don't think you are doing a good job with their child. Take some of the following sample comments:

> "My kid should be the starting pitcher in our playoff game, not Derrick. If you want to win that game, you should be starting my kid."

> "What's the deal with giving everyone all this playing time? My kid's the best player on the team, and he shouldn't be sitting out at all, unless it's a blowout."

> "What are you doing hitting my kid seventh in the lineup? He's a much better hitter than several of those players you've got ahead of him. He should be hitting third, if you ask me."

Well, you *didn't* ask that parent, and you didn't ask the other parents for their "advice," either. But sometimes you get it, free of charge.

Don't get into a long conversation with parents on how you coach their child. You don't need to defend your right to make coaching decisions. Tell parents politely and firmly that while you appreciate their concerns, those are coaching decisions reserved for you and any assistant coaches you might have. Remind them that the decisions you make are in the best interest of all the players, including their own son or daughter. And leave it at that.

Parents Who Yell at Umpires

If you've attended many youth baseball games, you've probably heard comments like the following:

> "C'mon, ump! He was safe by a mile!"

> "Hey, Blue! Want to borrow my glasses?"

> "That's terrible! This guy's strike zone changes every inning!"

Are parents justified in making derogatory or disparaging comments to or about umpires? Absolutely not, even if the ump misses the call. Youth league umpires are most often volunteers, unpaid and untrained. Yelling at the umpire is poor sporting behavior, and it sends the wrong message to kids:

> If I struck out, it was the umpire's fault. If we lost, it was because of lousy umpiring.

It tells kids it's okay to disrespect the umpire, it takes their focus off their own performance, and it implies that the game's outcome is far more important than it really is. It also usurps part of your role, which is to calmly discuss with umpires certain calls (these debates should be rare; you'll learn more about them in "Communicating with Opponents and Umpires," later in this chapter).

As noted earlier, let parents know up front what you expect of them, including their behavior at games. If they yell at the umpires during games, talk with them after the game. Perhaps call them a little later in the evening, after they've had time to cool off. Tell them you appreciate their support but that you need them to stop berating the umpires, even if they miss calls. Tell them why you feel this way (for the reasons stated in the previous paragraph), and ask that they refrain from doing so at future games.

Parents Who Yell at Their Own Kids

Parents who yell at their own kids—for striking out, for committing an error, for whatever reason—do a tremendous disservice to their children. The words of parents are extremely powerful, and they have the power to damage and destroy. Sadly, sports seem to be an arena in which some parents choose to harm their children's egos. Those damaging words reverberate in the youngster's ears long past the game and far from the field.

If a parent yells at his child during a game, counter the harmful words with your own words of encouragement and sincere praise. Just make sure the praise is truly sincere because kids can see through false praise and such praise can undermine your own credibility and their ability to believe you in this or other situations.

If you believe the situation warrants it, talk to that parent during the game or send a nonverbal message to him to cut the negative talk. Before doing this, though, consider whether you can send your message without fanning the flames on the spot. You don't want an escalated confrontation; you want the parent to stop yelling at his kid.

If you don't communicate with the parent on the spot, do so after the game, one on one. Tell the parent that his son needs his support and encouragement. If he can't provide that support and encouragement, ask the parent to stop attending games.

Parents Who Yell at Other Kids

Many parents cheer on their own kids but loudly disparage other players, either on their own child's team or on the opposing team. Take the following examples:

> "Hey, this kid can't hit! You're going to strike out, batter!"
>
> "Come on, left fielder, you should've had that ball!"
>
> "Hey, nice throw, shortstop!" (A comment made with dripping sarcasm.)

Don't tolerate this any more than you would tolerate parents verbally abusing their own child. Intervene in the same way you would with a parent yelling at her own son or daughter.

note

What you're trying to do in these situations is turn a win-lose situation into a win-win situation. You don't want to defeat parents; you want to win them over, so that you're on the same side, with the end result being that the players benefit.

Parents Who Abuse Their Children

Children can be abused physically, emotionally, and sexually. The signs of abuse are not always readily apparent, nor are they always easily separated from the scratches and bruises that come from normal childhood activity.

The point here is not to make you paranoid and suspect abuse when you see a player with a black eye, but to keep your own eyes open and watch for additional signs. Kids who are abused tend to

- Have a poor self-image
- Act out in practice or at games
- Be withdrawn, passive, or sad
- Lash out angrily at their peers

- Bully or intimidate weaker peers
- Have difficulty trusting others
- Be self-disparaging or self-destructive

Players who exhibit some or all of these signs might have been abused, or they might have experienced another child being abused. Complicating matters, these signs are also exhibited by kids who are undergoing various types of stress—for example, their parents' recent divorce.

If you do suspect that one of your players is being abused, it's your responsibility to contact the proper authorities—your local child protection services agency, police, hospital, or an emergency hotline. In many cases, you can do so anonymously. In any regard, if you have reason to believe abuse might be taking place, report it.

Communicating with League Administrators

Part of a league administrator's role is to set up and administer leagues. Administrators schedule games, set up league policies and rules, oversee the maintenance of the fields, dispense the necessary equipment, arrange for umpiring, and take care of many other responsibilities, all with the goal of providing a top-quality experience for the players.

A coach's interaction with league administrators generally falls into three categories:

- League information
- Coaches' meetings and clinics
- Questions and concerns

Let's look at each of these in the following sections.

League Information

The league should provide information on game schedules, practice field usage, equipment distribution, league policies and rules, and any upcoming coaches' meetings or clinics. Read the information you receive; make copies of the game schedules for parents; and talk with your administrator if you have any questions about the schedule, the policies, or any other information dispensed by the league.

Coaches' Meetings and Clinics

Most leagues hold a preseason coaches' meeting at which the administrator distributes the necessary information and updates coaches on new policies, modified rules, and other important matters.

Some leagues also conduct coaches' training. If your league offers such training, take advantage of it.

The point here is to consider ways to help you better prepare for your season. Coaching clinics and courses are one good way to do so.

Questions and Concerns

Take any overarching questions or concerns—about league policies or rules, practice field availability, scheduling, and so on—to your league administrator. In addition, if you have an ongoing problem with a parent and are unable to resolve it with that parent, consider talking with your league administrator. By all means, do so if the problem affects the enjoyment of the game for other fans, the parent poses some sort of physical threat to anyone, or the parent is verbally abusive at games and refuses to stop or leave when she becomes abusive.

tip

The American Sport Education Program (www.asep.com) offers effective training courses for youth coaches, including an online course in youth baseball. This is one of many good programs that can be found.

Communicating with Opponents and Umpires

Three key words here: *respect*, *dignity*, *restraint*.

Besides being your players' coach, you are also their role model, whether you like it or not. And how you communicate with opposing coaches, players, and umpires speaks volumes about what kind of role model you are.

If you have a question for an umpire, ask it at the proper time and without showing up the umpire or unnecessarily slowing the game. Treat the umpires, and the opposing coaches, with the same respect you'd like to be shown.

note

You can teach your kids all the requisite skills, but if you don't teach them how to play the game—all-out, having fun, and showing respect for the umpires and opponents—you haven't taught them enough.

At the ends of games, line up your players and lead them as you shake hands with the other team. Instruct your players to be respectful as they shake or slap hands. Also thank the umpires for volunteering their time.

THE ABSOLUTE MINIMUM

This chapter was all about what, when, and how to communicate with your players, parents, league administrators, opposing coaches and players, and umpires. Key points included

- Use the 10 keys to being a good communicator. Those keys are 1) Know your message; 2) Make sure you are understood; 3) Deliver your message in the proper context; 4) Use appropriate emotions and tones; 5) Adopt a healthy communication style; 6) Be receptive; 7) Provide helpful feedback; 8) Be a good nonverbal communicator; 9) Be consistent; and 10) Be positive.

- Contact parents before the season begins, sharing information about your coaching philosophy and practice and game schedules, and paving the way for healthy communication throughout the season.

- Let parents know what you expect of them, in terms of positive team support, and what they can expect of you.

- Suggest ways parents can be actively involved in supporting and helping the team.

- Work through the challenging situations parents sometimes present. Keep your players' best interests in mind as you work for win-win situations.

- If you have reason to believe a player has been abused, report it to local authorities.

- Give the umpires and opponents the same respect you would like to be shown. Be a model of good sporting behavior for your players.

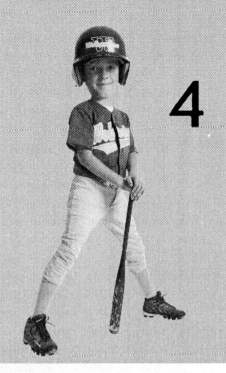

4

SAFETY PRINCIPLES

Baseball isn't a contact sport. But it is a sport that involves a lot of running, and collisions do happen. Add in balls that are thrown and hit, pitchers' arms that are wild, and young bodies that aren't always in complete control of themselves, and it's no wonder injuries occur in baseball.

Sometimes these injuries are preventable, and sometimes they aren't. This chapter focuses on how to create a safe environment for your players, provide the supervision they need, and do all you can to prevent injuries. You'll also learn how to respond to the injuries that do happen. Hopefully you won't have an emergency to respond to, but if you do, you need to know what action to take, so you'll learn about that as well. Finally, we'll consider safety precautions related to severe weather.

Communicating the Inherent Risks

Two outfielders converge on a fly ball, each yelling, "I got it, I got it!" As they collide, the only thing they get is a shiny goose egg to show for their efforts.

On a line drive up the middle, the pitcher can't get his glove up in time to protect himself; the ball zings him on the shoulder. A runner slides into second and sprains his knee. Sprinting to beat a throw to first, a batter/runner strains a hamstring. Another batter is hit on the hand by a pitch.

These are just some of the ways players get injured in baseball. Scrapes, cuts, bruises, muscle cramps and spasms, and muscle strains account for about two thirds of injuries in baseball; sprains, fractures, and other injuries also occur, though less frequently. Major injuries are rare, but they do occur. In comparison with other sports, baseball is among the leaders in eye injuries and accounts for nearly half of all sports-related mouth injuries.

One of the most common injuries in baseball is to pitchers' arms. Because of the strain placed on their arms, nearly half of all pitchers under age 12 have chronic elbow pain. You'll learn later how you can reduce the likelihood of pitching injuries.

Like all sports, baseball has its inherent risks. It's your duty to communicate these risks to parents. As mentioned in Chapter 3, "Communication Keys," you should do this before the season starts, either in a letter or in a parent meeting.

What should you say? Tell the parents about the types of injuries that can occur. Assure them that you will do all in your power to prevent injuries, but that you can't prevent all injuries, and parents and players should understand the risks going in.

Ask parents to do their part, meaning equipping their children with adequate footwear (rubber cleats are preferable to provide traction) and gloves that fit well. Let parents know you will do your part in providing adequate supervision at practices and games.

Many leagues have consent forms parents must fill out. In doing so, parents acknowledge that they understand the risks involved and do not hold the coach or the league liable for injuries that occur while players are participating in the program.

warning

Consent forms do not protect you from all liability issues. If you do not provide adequate supervision or respond appropriately to an injured player, you can still be held liable. However, by being able to prove that you provided proper supervision and instruction, you are less likely to be held accountable for a player's injury.

Being Prepared

There are several actions you can take to be prepared to handle injury and emergency situations. Three of those actions include

- Having CPR/first aid training
- Being prepared to respond to kids with chronic health conditions
- Having a well-stocked first aid kit on hand

Beyond these, you should also have a plan for responding to both minor injuries and major injuries. You'll learn more about those plans a little later in this chapter. For now, let's take a look at the three items just mentioned.

CPR/First Aid Training

CPR and first aid training is often offered through local hospitals and medical clinics, as well as through national organizations such as the American Red Cross. Sports leagues often sponsor or arrange for the training, which covers the basics of providing cardiopulmonary resuscitation and first aid for a variety of injuries.

If you have the opportunity to be trained in CPR/first aid, take it. Understanding the proper response and practicing the correct techniques involved go much further than reading about the topic.

If you don't have the opportunity to be trained, study this chapter carefully and supplement your learning with additional resources as you see fit.

Chronic Health Condition Awareness

Dontrelle legs out a double and then stands on second base, wheezing hard; he can't seem to catch his breath. His wheezing is beyond the normal out-of-breath, out-of-shape gasping for air. He is truly having trouble getting enough air into his lungs. What do you do?

Hannah is stung by a bee and her eyes begin to itch and swell. She develops hives and begins wheezing. How do you respond?

Tyler begins sweating and trembling. He is turning pale. You know he is diabetic. What action do you take?

Dontrelle has asthma, Hannah is allergic to bee stings, and Tyler (as mentioned) suffers from diabetes. These are examples of chronic conditions that some of your players might have and that you might have to deal with as your season progresses. With chronic health conditions, it's vital that you

■ Are aware that the child has the condition

■ Know the signs the child will exhibit when the condition is bothering him or her

■ Know how to respond to the symptoms

Before the first practice, have parents fill out a medical emergency form (see Appendix B, "Medical Emergency Form"). On this form they can note what type of allergy or condition their child has, which symptoms to watch for, what to do in case of an attack or episode, and at what phone numbers they can be reached.

If parents note an allergy or condition but are sparse with their information on what signs to look for, ask them directly what you should watch for. You can also find this information easily on the Internet or through resources in your library.

Just as important as knowing what to look for is knowing how to respond. The child's parents are the first and most important resource here; they will know what treatment is called for. Some situations will call for you to seek immediate emergency help. Know what these situations are and carry the appropriate medical emergency numbers—and a cell phone, if possible—with you at practices and games. If you don't have a cell phone, carry change with you for a pay phone.

First Aid Kit

Stock a first aid kit and take it with you to practices and games. Some stores sell complete kits; you can buy an already-assembled kit or put one together on your own. Either way, here are the essentials you should have on hand:

■ Phone numbers of parents, players' doctors, emergency medical personnel, and police

■ Change for a pay phone

■ Antiseptic wipes

■ Antibacterial soap

■ First aid cream

■ Instant cold pack

■ Gauze rolls

■ Triangular bandages

■ 2" elastic bandage

■ Bandages, sheer and flexible, of various sizes

■ Nonstick pads of assorted sizes

■ Hypoallergenic first aid tape

- Oval eye pads
- Acetaminophen
- Scissors
- Tweezers
- Insect sting kit
- Disposable gloves
- First aid guide
- Contents card

> **tip**
>
> Use the contents card to remind you of what you *should* have and what you *do* have, so you know when to restock. Use the first aid guide to help you remember how to care for minor injuries (it's easier than carrying this book with you to practice).

Providing Proper Supervision

In the rush to provide superior coaching and teaching, to shape their youngsters into the best possible baseball players over the course of a season, many coaches overlook an even more important duty: to provide proper supervision at practices and games.

Parents are entrusting their children to you; your most important duty is to make sure their kids are cared for and supervised in a safe environment.

To provide the supervision your players need, be sure you

- Plan your practices.
- Inspect the field and equipment.
- Provide proper instruction.
- Supervise each activity.

Plan Your Practices

In Chapter 5, "Practice Plans," you'll learn how to plan your season and individual practices. Planning prepares you to instruct and coach more effectively. When you're organized and know what you want to teach, and how you want to teach it, you're more likely to stay on task and maintain control. In turn, your players are more likely to stay focused, taking their cues from you, and less likely to have down time to fool around while you're figuring out what to do next.

You'll learn to plan your practices using a logical progression of skills, based on your players' level of development and physical condition.

Keep these season and practice plans; they can be important if an injury were to occur and your judgment in terms of planning were questioned. Also fill out and keep any injury reports (see Appendix C, "Injury Report") for your records.

Inspect the Field and Equipment

Check your practice and game fields before playing on them. Look for holes, broken glass, rocks, and other items—either part of the natural terrain or man-made—that pose a threat to your players. If there are hazards on the field that you can't remove or fix, do whatever you can to reduce the risks they present and warn your players about them. Then report those hazards to your league administrator.

Inspect the equipment your players use, as well. Make sure the catcher's gear is in good shape and that it fits the players who wear it. Also make sure your batting helmets are in good repair and that your players choose helmets that fit them.

Provide Proper Instruction

If a pitcher has no idea how to properly deliver a pitch, two players are at risk: the batter and the pitcher, the latter of whom is likely to injure his arm. Likewise, if fielders don't understand the techniques for fielding and baserunners don't know how to slide, injuries are much more likely to happen.

That's why it's so important that you teach your players the proper technique for all the skills they need to perform. It not only increases their chances of playing well, but also decreases their chances of being injured.

Nearly one third of baseball injuries result from sliding into bases. If players don't know the correct technique, they can sprain their ankles or get *strawberries* (abrasions) on their legs. Breakaway bases cut down on the number of sliding injuries, but many leagues don't use them. Regardless of the type of base your league uses, your players need to know how to slide correctly. You'll learn how to teach this skill in Chapter 9, "Offensive Skills and Tactics."

Supervise Each Activity

Planning the practice, knowing what you want your players to be doing from minute to minute, isn't enough. You need to closely supervise the players as they participate in each activity. Accidents and injuries are more likely to happen when activities are not supervised.

That means don't get kids started in an activity and then watch them out of the corner of your eye while you make a call on your cell phone. It also means not temporarily leaving the practice field, leaving the players in the charge of your teenage son. It means staying focused on the activity, being there to provide feedback on players' performances, and—most importantly from a legal standpoint—ensuring that the activity is conducted safely and that all players are under your direct supervision.

For additional ways to make practices safe, see the following sidebar, "Safety Tips."

SAFETY TIPS

Here are five more ways to provide for your players' safety:

- Remember that your players are kids, not miniature adults. Their bodies can't take the physical stress that adults' bodies can. Don't encourage kids to play through pain, and don't expect them to do what you can do.

- Stretch and warm up properly for practices and games. Lead your players through a warm-up routine that includes a few minutes of easy running followed by stretching leg, arm, and shoulder muscles. Instruct your players to make short and easy throws as they loosen up for practices and games and to gradually make the throws longer and harder as their arms warm up. Make sure your pitchers warm up adequately before they enter a game.

- Make clear rules pertaining to when and where players can swing bats and throw balls, and enforce the rules. Don't allow players to pick up a bat and take a practice cut wherever they are. They should be in the batter's box, in the on-deck circle, or under your direct supervision when they have a bat in their hands—and always with a helmet on. Don't allow players to pitch to each other "on the side"; you should directly supervise all live pitching and hitting. Institute similar types of rules for when and where players can throw balls. Supervise their throwing warm-ups so they throw in the same directional path. Talk about other safety rules as well: wearing a helmet while in the on-deck circle and on the bases, as well as while batting; the on-deck batter staying in the circle and watching the batter in case a foul ball is hit in her direction; the other players staying on the bench or in the dugout while their teammates bat; and so on.

- Handle your pitchers with care. Consider keeping a pitch count. In one recent study, kids from ages 9 to 12 who threw more than 75 pitches per game were 50% more likely to have elbow pain than kids who threw less than 25 pitches per game. Consider limiting your pitchers to no more than 75 pitches per game. An assistant or a parent volunteer could help you keep track of pitches.

- Don't allow pitchers to throw anything but fastballs. Why? Studies show that pitchers under age 12 who throw curves and sliders have an increased risk of elbow and shoulder pain. Even if they don't feel the pain immediately, their risk of future overuse injury is greater if they throw curves and sliders before they reach their teen years.

Responding to Minor Injuries

The focus so far has been on doing all you can to prevent injuries from occurring. Still, they will occur, and you need to know how to respond to them.

Most of the injuries in youth baseball are minor: cuts and scrapes, bruises, sprains, and strains. Here's how you should respond in each situation.

Cuts and Scrapes

Remember the disposable gloves in your first aid kit? Here's where you use them: as a barrier between you and a player's blood. While wearing the gloves, stop the bleeding by pressing directly on the cut with a gauze bandage. If the cut is deep enough that blood soaks the bandage, keep that bandage in place and apply another one.

When the bleeding has stopped, remove the gauze bandage and cleanse the wound with an antiseptic wipe. Apply some first aid cream. Then place a clean bandage over the wound.

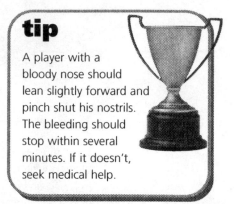

tip

A player with a bloody nose should lean slightly forward and pinch shut his nostrils. The bleeding should stop within several minutes. If it doesn't, seek medical help.

Bruises

Things sometimes go bump in the night. More often, they go bump at second base, in the outfield, or at home plate. Wherever the bump takes place, a bruise often results. Many bruises don't need any special treatment, but if the area is swollen and tender, treat it through the PRICE method:

tip

Apply ice for about 15 minutes every 3 hours or so during the day. When the swelling decreases, the player can begin gentle range-of-motion exercises for the affected joint.

- **P = Protect**—Keep the athlete from further harm as you tend to the injury.

- **R = Rest**—This hastens the healing process.

- **I = Ice**—This reduces inflammation in the injured area, which aids in the healing process; it also reduces the pain.

- **C = Compress**—When you compress the injured area with a tightly secured ice bag (use an elastic bandage to do this), you ensure that the ice can do its job.

- **E = Elevate**—When you raise the injured area above the heart level, this minimizes the amount of blood that pools in the area. The more blood that pools in the area, the longer the injury will take to heal.

Sprains and Strains

A *sprain* happens when ligaments or tendons are stretched too far from their normal position. Typically, a sprain occurs in the ankle, knee, or wrist. A sprain generally causes pain, swelling, and bruising of the affected joint.

A *strain* occurs when a muscle is stretched too far. In baseball, the most common strains are to hamstrings (the muscles in the backs of the thighs) and shoulder muscles. A strained hamstring generally relates to a single, specific incident (for example, sprinting to first base), while a shoulder strain is usually a repetitive, overuse injury, suffered most often by pitchers.

Treat sprains and strains with the PRICE method. The player should fully recover and gradually work back to full speed.

Remember to use the injury report to keep a record of all injuries, including minor ones.

> **note**
>
> Overuse injuries result from the stress placed on bodies by repetitive training. Such injuries can include stress fractures, strains, sprains, tendonitis, bursitis, and shin splints.

RETURNING AFTER AN INJURY

Most players want to return from an injury as soon as possible. But if they return too quickly, they can aggravate the injury and end up missing more action than necessary.

Here are some guidelines for when injured players can return to action:

- They should return when they have been cleared to do so by their parents and, if appropriate, by their doctor.
- They should not practice or play if they still feel pain in the injured area during rest.
- They should use simple exercises to gently work the injured area once they have no pain at rest.
- If they feel pain as they resume exercising, they should stop.
- They should return gradually to full intensity, listening to their bodies and increasing intensity only when they can do so without pain.

Responding to Emergency Situations

You need to be prepared to respond to emergency situations such as broken bones and head, neck, and back injuries. An emergency situation can also crop up with a chronic health condition. Your role here is not to treat the player, but to facilitate that treatment while protecting the player from further harm.

To do so, you need to have an emergency plan in place. Here are the essentials of such a plan:

1. Evaluate the player and use your CPR/first aid training as appropriate. However, do *not* move, or allow the movement of, a player who has suffered a neck or back injury, a dislocated joint, or a broken bone.

2. Contact medical personnel, reassure the child, keep others away from him, and remain with the child until medical help arrives. Assign an assistant coach or a parent to call medical personnel, if possible. It's ideal that you stay with the player, to keep him calm.

3. If the child is taken to the hospital and his parents are not available to go with him, appoint an assistant coach or a parent to accompany the child. Ideally, this person will be someone the player knows and can take comfort from.

> **tip**
>
> Always carry these phone numbers with you at practices and games: players' parents (home, office, and mobile phones), players' physicians, hospital, police, and rescue unit. Also be sure you have players' emergency information on hand. You'll gain this information through the form found in Appendix B, "Medical Emergency Form."

Heatstroke

In heatstroke, a person's body temperature climbs dangerously high as heat is generated more quickly than the body can handle it. As the body's thermoregulatory mechanisms fail, heatstroke can occur. In the late stages of heatstroke, the person loses his ability to sweat, but this isn't the case earlier on.

Signs of heatstroke include

- Fatigue and weakness
- Nausea and vomiting
- Headache
- Dizziness
- Muscle cramps
- Irritability

A person suffering from heatstroke has hot, flushed skin. He likely also has a rapid pulse, shallow breathing, and constricted pupils. The person might exhibit strange behavior and confusion.

What should you do if a player exhibits some of these signs? Get the player into shade, have him sit or lie down, remove any excess clothing or equipment, and cool his body with wet towels or by pouring cold water over him. Have someone call medical personnel immediately. Have the player drink cool water. Another way to cool the body is to place ice packs on the armpits, neck, and back and between the legs.

Under no circumstances should you allow an athlete who has suffered heatstroke to return to action until he has been examined by a doctor and cleared to play.

Heat Exhaustion

Heat exhaustion happens when a person becomes dehydrated. This person usually is sweating profusely and has pale, clammy skin; a rapid and weak pulse; dilated pupils; and a loss of coordination.

The signs of heat exhaustion are the same as for heatstroke. The treatment is also the same, with the exception that you might not need to send for medical personnel. Send for medical personnel if the player's condition doesn't improve or if it worsens. Again, don't let the player resume practicing or playing without the consent of her physician.

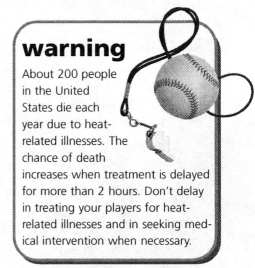

warning

About 200 people in the United States die each year due to heat-related illnesses. The chance of death increases when treatment is delayed for more than 2 hours. Don't delay in treating your players for heat-related illnesses and in seeking medical intervention when necessary.

Respecting the Weather

The weather can present significant threats to the well-being of players and coaches. In this section, you'll learn about guidelines for three weather-related situations: heat, lightning, and severe weather.

Heat Guidelines

Heatstroke and heat exhaustion most commonly occur in hot, humid weather. To help prevent heat illnesses, use caution in hot climates. Here are some guidelines for exercising in the heat:

- Realize it takes a week or two for the body to adapt to a hot environment. That means if you've had a cool spring and suddenly a heat wave strikes, the heat will affect your players more in that first week or two.
- When it's hot, train before 10 a.m. or after 4 p.m. if at all possible.
- Wear loose-fitting, light-colored clothing because it's coolest and allows more sweat to evaporate.
- Encourage your players to drink water before they come to practice, and have water on hand at practice. You might suggest that your players bring their own water bottles. They should drink about 4–6 ounces of water every 20

minutes in hot or humid conditions. Tell them to drink plenty of water after practice as well.

■ On hot or humid days, take a 5- to 10-minute water break in the middle of practice. Get in the shade while you do so.

Lightning Guidelines

Your league might have lightning guidelines in place; if so, follow those. If not, use the *flash-to-bang method* to determine your response. After you see a flash of lightning, begin counting seconds. Stop counting when you hear thunder. For every 5 seconds you count, the lightning is 1 mile away. So, if you count 10 seconds, the lightning is 2 miles away; if you count 15 seconds, the lightning is 3 miles away; and so on.

You should take immediate defensive action when lightning is indicated within 6–8 miles (30–40 "flash-to-bang" seconds). Why? Because the next bolt of lightning can strike 6–8 miles away from the previous strike. Don't be fooled into thinking it's far away; *it isn't*.

When lightning is within 6–8 miles, do the following:

■ Stop playing or practicing. Seek shelter immediately inside a safe structure (one with four walls). Dugouts are not safe shelters. The safest shelters have electrical and telephone wiring as well as plumbing because these aid in grounding the structure.

■ If you cannot find such a shelter, a fully enclosed vehicle with a metal roof is your next best choice. The windows should be completely closed. It is important that you not touch any part of the metal framework of the vehicle while inside it as the storm is occurring.

■ Avoid high points in open fields. Don't stand under or near trees, flagpoles, or light poles.

If you feel your hair stand on end, feel your skin tingle, or hear crackling noises, assume the lightning safety position. Crouch on the ground with your weight on the balls of your feet. Keep your feet together, lower your head, and cover your ears. Do *not* lie flat on the ground.

note

It *is* okay to use a cell phone during a thunderstorm. However, it is *not* advisable to use a landline phone.

Severe Weather Guidelines

Don't hold practice if there is a tornado or severe weather watch or warning for your area. If a tornado or severe storm watch or warning comes up after you have begun practice or a game, seek immediate shelter in the nearest building.

If no buildings are nearby, the next best thing is to head for the lowest ground, preferably in a ditch or ravine. If a bridge or highway overpass is nearby, it can offer shelter as well. Get as close as you can to the top and hold tightly to the supports.

Unlike the protection they can offer to those trying to avoid lightning, cars are one of the worst places you can be with a tornado approaching.

THE ABSOLUTE MINIMUM

This chapter is intended to prepare you to provide for the safety of your players. Among the main points are these:

- Let parents know of the inherent risks of playing baseball before the season begins.

- There are many ways you can prepare yourself to provide for safety. Among them are being trained in CPR/first aid, being aware of any chronic health conditions of your players, knowing how to respond if a player's health condition flares up, and having a well-stocked first aid kit on hand at all practices and games.

- One of your most important duties is to provide proper supervision at practices and games. This comes through planning your practices, inspecting the field and equipment, providing proper instruction, and closely supervising each activity.

- Know how to respond to minor injuries, including cuts and scrapes, bruises, and sprains and strains.

- Have an emergency plan in place, have all the important phone numbers you need in case of an emergency, and enact the plan when a major injury happens.

- Respect the weather. Know the guidelines for exercising in the heat and be aware of the symptoms of heat illness and how you should respond to it. Also know the guidelines for taking cover when lightning or severe weather is in the area.

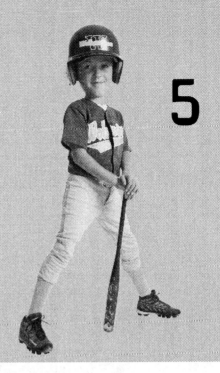

5

PRACTICE PLANS

Generally, the people who volunteer their time—such as for coaching—are already busy people. Now they add one more thing to their plate. And then, in the few quiet moments of their day (usually lasting no more than 30 seconds), they wonder how they are going to find the time to fulfill their latest volunteer obligations.

Many inexperienced coaches, pressed for time and unaware of the harm they are doing, go into and through the season winging it from practice to practice. Their argument is simple: They don't have the time to prepare.

You don't need to spend massive amounts of time in preparation for your season and practices. But spending some preparation time will greatly aid your coaching efforts.

So, use this chapter to help you prepare for your season and your practices. You will be glad you did—and your players will be, too. Your practices will run more smoothly, with less down time. Your players will learn all they need to learn, and in a logical order. And you will get the most out of your limited time with your players.

Planning Your Season

If you plan from practice to practice without keeping the big picture in mind, you risk overlooking some tactics or skills you should be teaching; you also risk presenting the skills you do teach in less than an ideal order. To make an extreme example, it's no good teaching your players the hit-and-run before they know how to hit. It's equally pointless to focus on double plays before your players can field grounders and make good throws to the proper base. When you develop a season plan, consider what you should teach throughout the season and when you should teach it.

These three elements will help you construct a plan for your season:

- Purpose
- Tactics and skills
- Rules

Purpose

You should have an overall purpose for every practice, and, when considered in context of the entire season, there should be a logical flow to the purpose of each practice. For example, the purposes in the early-season practices should be to introduce and teach the basic skills. As the season progresses, the purposes should become to refine the basic skills and learn the tactics related to those skills (and to learn more complex skills, if appropriate for the age you're coaching).

Having a purpose gives the practice an informed drive and energy. You and your players are there for a particular reason that day, and your time is spent in trying to accomplish the goals for that practice.

Tactics and Skills

Based on the purpose of the practice, you will focus on teaching a particular skill or tactic. That doesn't mean your players don't practice other tactics or skills during that practice, but that the main emphasis is on learning or refining a particular skill or tactic.

When you lay out, in a season plan, all the skills and tactics you plan to teach, it helps to ensure that you don't overlook something important and that your teaching has a logical flow.

Rules

Many coaches overlook teaching rules to their players. Don't assume your players know the rules. Plan to take some time to teach the basic rules; your players need to know these as much as they need to develop their skills. When you make plans to teach the basic rules, you're much more likely to take the time to do so.

> **tip**
>
> Teach rules within the context of playing. Set up a tag-up baserunning situation, briefly explain and demonstrate the rule, and then practice it. Players learn rules much better in an action context, as opposed to you simply telling them the rules.

Adjusting Your Season Plan

If you are coaching 6- and 7-year-olds, your season plan will be simpler than if you were coaching 9- and 10-year-olds. As kids gain in size, experience, and physical abilities, they are able to learn more advanced skills and tactics. In general, keep your plans simple and adjust them as you need to based on your players' abilities. If they've demonstrated they have picked up the basics more quickly than you thought they would, step up your plans a bit. For example, if your 9- and 10-year-olds have demonstrated that they can pretty consistently field ground balls and make force plays, take the next step of working on executing double plays. If, on the other hand, you had planned to work on double plays by midseason and your players still haven't mastered fielding grounders and making good throws, keep your focus on developing those more fundamental skills before moving on to the double play. And it might be that you never do move on to the double play that season.

The main point is to adjust your plan to what the players need.

Sample Season Plan

Table 5.1 contains a sample 8-week season plan for a 9- and 10-year-old team that meets once a week. Use it as a guide when you construct your own season plan. Appendix D, "Season Plan," has a blank season plan you can use.

Create your season plan before the season begins. Construct a plan that reflects however many times you will practice throughout the season. Plan your season the way you believe will work best for your players, so long as you cover the basics first and move at a pace that is good for them, adjusting as need be.

Note that although you have one main purpose, or focus, you can and should work on multiple skills in a single practice. This model is *not* meant to be the one-and-only way to plan your season; it is one example, intended to give you a start.

TABLE 5.1   8-week Practice Plan

Week	Purpose	Tactics/Skills	Rules
1	Catching and throwing	Catching technique Throwing technique Hitting technique	What's a catch and what's a trapped ball
2	Fielding ground balls and fly balls	Fielding ground balls, making throws to first Catching pop-ups in the infield and fly balls in the outfield Hitting practice Running through first base Sliding	Infield fly rule Running past first base Defensive and offensive interference Your league's sliding rules
3	Throwing to the proper base	Fielding ground balls and fly balls in the infield and outfield; making throws to the proper base Blocking the plate Hitting practice Running the bases Tag-up plays for the baserunner	Tagging up after a catch Your league lead-off and stealing rules
4	Making force plays and tag plays	Executing force outs Executing tag plays Hitting practice Tag-up plays for the baserunner	Force-out rule Tag play rule
5	Making the double play	Executing double plays	Offensive and defensive interference rules
6	Review and refine	Practice the fielding skills most needed Hitting practice	
7	Review and refine	Practice the fielding skills most needed Hitting practice	
8	Review and refine	Practice the fielding skills most needed Hitting practice	

Planning Practices

After you have your season plan in place, you can begin to construct your practice plans. Create your practice plans one at a time—that is, don't create your entire season's worth of practice plans at once because you might find you need to adjust them based on what your players need most to focus on.

This section covers the essential structure of your practices; in a later section, "12 Keys to Conducting Effective Practices," we delve into the methods that will help you run successful practices within the structure presented here.

The Best Option: Simultaneous Stations

Baseball coaches have two basic options in structuring their practices. One option is to have all the players together, receiving instruction and then practicing the skills and tactics in one large group. Advantages to this option are that all the players receive the exact same instruction and the coach can easily view the action and provide feedback because only one station is being used. The downfall is that practice time isn't being maximized; players are standing around, waiting for their turn to hit or field or run the bases. With only one ball in play and about 15 players, that's an inefficient way to practice. Players learn and develop their skills less and have more time to goof off.

The better option is to run simultaneous stations. After a team warm-up, split the team into three groups and set up three stations. After every 15 minutes, instruct each group to rotate to a new station. By the end of practice, each group will have had 15 minutes at each of the three stations. (With a 5- to 10-minute warm-up and a 5-minute wrap-up, that makes for a 60-minute practice.) In this way, players are active and engaged, they receive more chances to improve their skills, and they're having more fun.

What stations you set up depend on what you are focusing on. Figures 5.1 and 5.2 show two examples of setting up three-station fields.

FIGURE 5.1

Plan one for three-station practices.

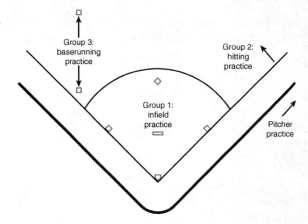

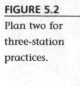

FIGURE 5.2
Plan two for
three-station
practices.

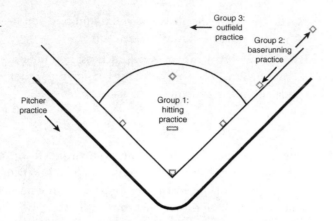

In Figure 5.1, group 1 begins with infield practice; group 2 begins with hitting practice; and group 3 practices baserunning. In Figure 5.2, group 1 begins with hitting practice; group 2 begins with baserunning practice; and group 3 begins with outfield practice. Again, in each instance, the groups rotate after 15 minutes.

In both cases, a pitcher and catcher (a volunteer parent could be the catcher) could practice near a sideline in foul territory, or outside the field, if there is room and you can safely supervise them while they are outside the field.

Simultaneous situations can provide the best learning experiences for players and make practices more active and fun, but they can also present challenges. You need to be aware of those challenges and know how to overcome them. There are two primary challenges: ensuring player safety and maintaining the quality of instruction and feedback provided to players.

Player Safety

Player safety, with simultaneous stations, can be at risk for two reasons: lack of adequate space for setting up the stations and lack of adequate adult supervision. Simply put, don't set up simultaneous stations if you feel that space limitations or lack of supervision will compromise your players' safety.

Set up your stations in a way that allows the players at each station to not be infringed upon by play from another station. The station that can present the most concern here is the hitting station. Wherever you set up this station, make sure you have *shaggers* (fielders) ready to field the ball near any other station that a hitter might be able to reach or hit toward. Also have a shagger who can protect either the pitcher or the catcher—whichever player has her back turned to the hitting station.

As for supervision, the ideal is to have one adult per station. When you include the pitcher throwing on the side (refer to Figures 5.1 and 5.2), that means four adults.

Do you *need* four adults to safely supervise simultaneous stations? No. Some experienced coaches have safely run simultaneous stations by themselves. In this case, you would set up each station, get players going in each, and move from station to station, observing and providing feedback.

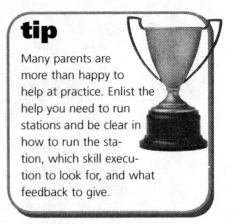

tip

Many parents are more than happy to help at practice. Enlist the help you need to run stations and be clear in how to run the station, which skill execution to look for, and what feedback to give.

In a better scenario, you will have an assistant coach. (If an assistant hasn't been assigned to you, ask the parents of your players if one or more would like to assist you. Generally, at least one parent will offer to help.) The setup time for the stations is quicker with an assistant available, and one coach can watch two stations while the other watches the third.

In the best scenario, you will have an assistant coach and some parent volunteers who can aid in watching and running stations. In this way, you could have an adult at each station providing feedback.

If you have an assistant coach and no other volunteers, you should still be able to run simultaneous stations. The drawback is you can't provide all the feedback you'd like because you can't be two places at once. You move from station to station, and you can be at one station and observe some of the action from another station, or you can stand between two stations and observe much of the action from both, but it's not the same as being at one station, focused only on the players and the action there.

But it's still worth it because the players get more skill practice this way. You just have to make sure you provide the instruction and feedback they need.

Coaching Instruction and Feedback

Of course, the primary purpose of the simultaneous stations is to give players more practice at skill execution. But if Damon continually moves his head and "steps in the bucket" (moves his lead foot toward third base as a right-handed hitter) as he practices hitting, is he going to improve his hitting skills? Not likely.

Players need feedback on their skill execution. They need to know what's right, what's wrong, and how to fix what's wrong. It's that feedback that helps them learn and improve.

When you have a coach or parent volunteer at each station, you are in the best situation for providing that feedback. Realize, however, that many parents might not know precisely what to look for or what feedback to provide; tell any volunteer exactly what to look for and what type of feedback to give. Give volunteers the easier stations to run, in terms of providing feedback. The baserunning station should be the simplest to supervise.

Sample Practice Plan

In Appendix E you'll find a blank practice plan you can photocopy and use. See Figure 5.3 for a sample 60-minute practice plan.

Here are a few things to note about the sample plan:

note

Some skills—specifically, making cutoff throws from the outfield and throwing from the outfield directly to a base—require the entire field. When practicing such plays, plan a full-field station for the beginning or end of practice.

- Instruction time is allotted for each of the stations. You won't always need to allot time for instruction, though. If you have already instructed your players on the skill or tactic, you can start the station with a drill or game.

- Most of the time at a station should be spent in games or drills. You'll learn more about setting up games and drills in "12 Keys to Conducting Effective Practices."

- The Comments section is meant for you to write coaching tips and technique reminders that you want to focus on in that station.

- The Notes section is for things you observe as the players perform at each station. Use this section to jot down observations you want to bring up at the end of practice or techniques you want to work on at the next practice. Use this section to keep a log or journal on each player's progress.

Conducting Your First Practice

Your first practice is different from all the other practices in a few respects. First, you're probably meeting the majority of your players for the first time, so introductions are in order. Second, you want to create, at the outset, the proper environment, one that balances fun with learning. Your players need to understand that you're there to help them learn and improve their skills. They also need to know what to expect from you and what you expect from them.

You can accomplish this in relatively short order—probably taking 5–10 minutes. From there, you can conduct your practice as normal.

FIGURE 5.3

A 60-minute practice plan.

Sample Practice Plan

Date <u>June 15</u>   Place <u>McKenzie Field</u>   Time <u>5:30 p.m.</u>

Equipment <u>2 extra bases/extra home plate/bats/balls/helmets</u>

Purpose <u>Infield defense: fielding grounders, throwing to first base</u>

Activity	Description	Time	Comments
1. Warm-up	Run, stretch, throw	5-10 min	Focus them on practice purpose
2a. STATION 1: FIELDING	*Instruction:* Fielding ground balls, making throws to first base	5 min	Move to the ball. Watch ball in glove. Skip and throw.
	Game: "Grounder Gobblers"	10 min	5 gounders per player. Keep track of overall team score.
2b. STATION 2: HITTING	*Instruction:* Hitting technique	5 min	Transfer weight from back to front. Swing parallel through zone. Head still.
	Practice: "10 and out"	10 min	10 swings, then rotate within group.
2c. STATION 3: BASERUNNING	*Instruction:* Sliding	5 min	Begin slide 10-12 feet from bag. Form figure "4" with legs. Extended foot slightly off the ground.
	Game: "Throw 'em out"	10 min	Rotate runners; 4-5 slides each in tag play situtation.
3. Wrap-up		5 min	Instructional reminders. Next practice reminder.

Notes

Need more work on getting in front of ball. Also on making good strong throw to first.

Some hitters are pulling their heads away, bailing out on pitch.

Structure your first practice like this:

1. **Introduction (5–10 minutes)**—Coach and player introductions (kids enjoy a fun icebreaker game here). Goals for the season. Your expectations of players and what they can expect of you. The practice structure. Team rules and safety issues. See the following sidebar, "Setting the Tone," for more detail on this first-practice introduction.

2. **Warm-up (5–10 minutes)**—Light running, stretching, throwing.

3. **Station 1 (10–15 minutes)**—Fielding ground balls instruction and practice. Situational plays.

4. **Station 2 (10–15 minutes)**—Fielding fly balls instruction and practice. Situational plays.

5. **Station 3 (10–15 minutes)**—Hitting instruction and practice.

6. **Wrap-up (5 minutes)**—Reinforce what most needs to be reinforced, based on activities. Remind players of the next practice or game.

SETTING THE TONE

To get off on the right foot, you need to communicate certain messages in the first practice and set the tone for a good learning environment. Some things to consider covering in that first practice are

- **Goals for the season**—Briefly tell players your goals for the season, which should be centered on helping them improve their skills, increase their understanding of the game, and have fun.

- **Your expectations**—Let them know that you expect them to show up on time for practice, to pay attention to your instruction and feedback, to obey any rules you set up (mainly concerned with safety), to give full effort, to respect others, to ask questions if they don't understand something, to ask for help when they need it, and to tell you if they are hurt.

- **What players can expect**—Also let players know what to expect from you: that you're there to provide instruction, feedback, and encouragement, to help each player improve his or her skills.

- **Practice structure**—Briefly let players see the big picture of how a typical practice will go.

- **Team rules/safety issues**—Inform players of your rules regarding swinging bats, throwing balls, and wearing helmets. Also talk about dugout or bench protocol (or you might address this prior to the first game). Don't go overboard on rules, but do be clear about safety issues and be strict in enforcing them.

Keep this meeting short, but don't skip over it.

---

12 Keys to Conducting Effective Practices

To this point you've learned about structuring your season and individual practices. The rest of this chapter is devoted to detailing 12 keys to running effective practices. Here are the keys:

1. Be prepared.
2. Set the stage.
3. Involve parents.
4. Be active.
5. Be active with a purpose.
6. Make it fun.
7. Provide instruction.
8. Give feedback.
9. Be encouraging and supportive.
10. Promote teamwork and camaraderie.
11. Discipline players as necessary.
12. Wrap up the practice.

1. Be Prepared

Sixty minutes—or however long you have for practice—goes by quickly. If you go into practice unprepared, it will go by inefficiently, too.

A little preparation can go a long way. Plan your practice, know what you need to teach, how you want to teach it, which stations you want to run, and which drills or games you want to use to help your players practice their skills. Choose effective drills and games to maximize the learning experience. Be prepared to instruct, give feedback, and provide encouragement.

That doesn't mean you can't adjust or deviate from your plan. It means you have a plan you can adjust as you need to.

2. Set the Stage

You need to not only have a plan, but also let your players in on that plan. It helps them focus when they know what they're going to practice that day. Let them know the purpose of each practice and the purpose of each drill or game at the practice stations.

How you approach the practice greatly influences your players. If you are cavalier or seemingly uncaring about what happens at practice, your players will follow suit. If you are focused and positive and have a purpose in mind, your players will be more tuned in to the drills and games.

Another way you set the stage is in teaching skills. Don't simply teach the mechanics; let players know why they need to perform the skill, and in what type of situation they will be called upon to perform it in a game. You'll learn more about this in Chapter 6, "Player Development."

3. Involve Parents

Studies show that the more parents are involved in their kids' education, the better their kids do. This shouldn't be too surprising.

Parental involvement has the same effect on youth sport programs, too. But some coaches ward off parents, discouraging their participation. Why? Perhaps because the coaches fear they will lose control of the team when other adults step in or the coaches are concerned that their own lack of knowledge or coaching ability will be revealed. And then there are the few bad-apple parents who are know-it-alls or poor sports or who *do* want to impose their own will at practice. Coaches already have plenty to contend with and can't be blamed for not wanting to deal with this type of parent.

But coaches who steer clear of parental involvement miss out on the advantages that can come with involving them. Here are a few of the roles parents can serve:

- **Official or unofficial assistant coaches**—It's extremely helpful to have at least one assistant coach. As noted earlier, it's also helpful to have an adult, whether you call him or her an assistant coach or a parent aid or whatever, to supervise each station you run at practice. Parents can be shaggers for the hitting station, protecting players at the other stations from hit balls. They can be base coaches during games. They can even help you instruct, if they know the skill and know how to teach it.

- **Scorekeepers**—Keeping the scorebook during games is another way parents can help.

tip

Some parents want to help but can't do so at every practice or game. Make it easy for these parents to help by setting up a parent helper rotation. Come up with the ways you need help, find out how many parents are willing to provide that type of help, and set up a rotation for practices and games, so the burden is light and shared.

- **Drink and snack providers**—Set up a rotation for parents to provide drinks and snacks for games.
- **Special-event planners**—Ask a parent to organize any special event—a pizza party or swimming party—held during the season or for a postseason celebration.

4. Be Active

Baseball practices run the risk of being run in a way that leaves most players standing around most of the time. That's why you are encouraged to use simultaneous stations. Kids can't improve if they have to wait for 14 teammates to swing the bat or field the ball before they get a chance. Keep things moving at practice.

5. Be Active with a Purpose

But don't mistake movement and action with purpose. The next worst thing to kids standing around in practice doing nothing is kids bouncing all around the field like balls in a pinball machine with no purpose at all.

When you have prepared for the practice, and when you have set the stage for it and for the games and drills the players are getting ready to participate in, then the players' actions are guided by a unified purpose. And when they're guided by that purpose, they are better prepared to learn and hone their skills.

6. Make It Fun

You can have a plan, and you can have a purpose to that plan, but if the practice is dull and boring, filled with repetitive drills that don't seem connected to the actual sport of baseball, then you're in trouble. Kids won't pay attention, they won't learn, and they won't care because they're not having fun.

Remember in Chapter 1, "Your Coaching Approach," when you learned about the reasons kids play baseball? The biggest reason they play is that they want to have fun.

Your goal is to teach your players baseball. Their goal is to have fun. When you make your teaching fun, everyone wins.

How do you make practices fun? You've already read about the main way: Keep the kids active. But there's another ingredient, too.

That ingredient is this: Don't practice skills by doing boring, repetitive drills. Practice skills in game-like conditions. This makes it more exciting for your players—and when they need to perform those skills in real games, they'll be more apt to succeed because they've been executing in those same situations in practice. In addition, kids understand the concept of tactics much better when those tactics are introduced and practiced in the context of real-game situations.

Read more about this concept in the following sidebar, "Using Game-like Situations in Practice."

USING GAME-LIKE SITUATIONS IN PRACTICE

Consider ways you could teach the force out at second base. You could hit ground ball after ground ball to your infielders, having them make the throw to second base. Each ground ball you could hit directly at the infielder, not too hard, not too soft, not too high, not too low. The infielder would wait for the ball to come to her, scoop it up, and toss it to her teammate covering second.

And everyone would yawn, including the fielders involved. Is it practicing the force out? Yes. Is it boring beyond belief? Yes.

What could you do to make it more game-like? For starters, place a baserunner on first base and have him attempt to beat the throw to second. Then, instead of hitting five straight easy ground balls to your second baseman, spray the grounders around the infield, without letting the fielders know where you're going to hit. And *don't* always hit them directly at the fielder; batters in games certainly won't. Make the fielders move to their right, to their left. Make them charge the ball. Make them field short hops and in-between hops. Test them.

If you do, they'll be much more likely to pass the test in real games. And they'll have a lot more fun in practice preparing for the games.

But don't stop there. Kids love contests, games within games. So make a contest of your fielding games. Assign teams, or keep point totals for each group of players that rotates to the fielding station. Give them some incentives.

In other words, make it *fun*.

Be creative. Put kids in game-like situations for all the skills and tactics they practice. When you do, you're doing everyone—including yourself—a favor.

---

7. Provide Instruction

The next three items on this list—instruction, feedback, and encouragement—are foundational elements in coaching at practice and are closely, and often sequentially, related.

Most coaches realize that to run an effective practice they need to provide quality instruction for their players. But providing good instruction isn't necessarily easy; it's accomplished through a set of learned skills. You'll learn about how to be an effective instructor and teacher of skills in Chapter 6.

8. Give Feedback

After you instruct your players, your coaching duties have just begun. As your players practice the tactics and skills you've taught them, you need to observe their play, assess their technique and understanding, and give them feedback on anything they're doing wrong and on what they should do to improve. How to provide this feedback is also covered in Chapter 6.

9. Be Encouraging and Supportive

All players—from youth leagues through the major leagues—need encouragement and support. Baseball is a difficult and challenging game. The skills of the game are not easy to acquire, and even once acquired, they are not easy to consistently execute. A major league hitter is among the best hitters if he gets a hit 3 out of every 10 times to the plate; a major league catcher is very good if he can throw out 4 of 10 would-be base-stealers; and a major league pitcher is considered good if he gives up four earned runs per nine innings.

Think of it this way: On every play in a game, someone succeeds—and someone fails. A batter fails to get a hit, or a pitcher fails to get an out, or a defender fails to make a play, or a baserunner fails to advance.

Your players will struggle with picking up the basic skills and with consistently executing them. All players will struggle to improve, regardless of their skill level. You need to nurture their improvement with encouragement and provide a supportive environment for them, and the practice field is the place where this happens. You'll learn specifics of how to provide this encouragement in Chapter 6.

10. Promote Teamwork and Camaraderie

Baseball is a team game. Home runs and strikeouts grab attention, but a nifty force out at second or a well-placed sacrifice bunt can be just as crucial to a game's outcome. Is your home-run hitting outfielder, who gives up more runs through his errors than he creates with his bat, more valuable than your singles-hitting second baseman who makes all the plays in the field and consistently moves runners over? For that matter, can a *good*-fielding home-run hitter win games all by himself?

The teams that win more often than not are generally more fundamentally sound than other teams. They make a greater percentage of the plays in the field; they move the runners along with base hits or with outs to the right side of the field; they make throws to the correct base and hit the cutoff man. They know what to do, and more often than not, they are able to do it. They have players up and down the lineup who contribute to the win.

One of the joys of playing sports is the camaraderie players experience with their teammates. This occurs as players struggle together, as they pull for each other, as they go through wins and losses together, as they exult over individual successes and encourage each other in individual failures, all the while reinforcing the notion that those individual successes and failures are all part of a team effort.

That's how the game and the relationships between players *should* be viewed, and that's the environment you should cultivate. Here are a couple of ideas for cultivating it:

- At the beginning of the season, you or a player's parents could host a pizza and movie night. The players could get together, eat pizza, and watch a baseball movie, such as *Sandlot* or *Field of Dreams*.

- At the end of each practice, say something positive about each player. Don't force this; it has to be sincere. If it's too much to say something about every player, single out half of them for compliments at one practice, and address the other half of the team at the end of the next practice. "Way to hit the cutoff man, Jake," "Nice hitting today, Ramon," and "You were picking them up at short today, Michelle," are examples of the things you might say. When players hear you say something good about everyone, most often for doing small things correctly, it reinforces the team concept.

- Set up a buddy system at practice. Pair up players at each practice and ask that each player pick out something good that his partner did during practice. Switch buddies at each practice so kids get used to encouraging and complimenting different teammates. Again, this exchange shouldn't be forced; emphasize that you want the players to look for good things their teammates do and encourage them to continue to improve.

The main point is to look for ways to emphasize the team aspects of the game and cultivate an environment in which the support and encouragement doesn't just flow from coach to players, but from player to player as well.

11. Discipline Players As Necessary

Part of running an effective practice is to take care of any discipline problems that arise, so they don't disrupt the practice.

Even when you conduct a practice that keeps the players active through fun and meaningful drills and games, some kids might misbehave. Here are some suggestions for dealing with different types of misbehavior:

- **Minor misbehavior**—Many times you can ignore minor misbehavior, so long as it doesn't disrupt the practice or distract others from hearing you or from practicing. Kids will sometimes clown around or goof off to draw attention; sometimes if you ignore that behavior, the child will stop it without being told to. If the child *doesn't* stop it and it becomes a distraction to others, you should put a stop to it.

- **Disrespect**—When a player shows disrespect, either to you or to another player, don't let it pass. Use appropriate measures to stop the disrespect.

- **Repeated misbehavior**—If a player is repeatedly misbehaving, even if it's minor misbehavior, you need to address this. Talk to the player, tell him what behavior you need from him, and if the misbehavior continues, punish him appropriately. You might also want to call his parents to let them know of the problem and work together to steer the child toward good behavior.

- **Behavior that puts someone in danger**—You need to put an immediate stop to any behavior that puts someone in danger, and you need to discipline the misbehaving player accordingly.

When you do need to discipline players, do so consistently and impartially. Stick to what you say; if you tell them they will be disciplined for a certain type of behavior, and you don't follow through, you're in for trouble.

After you have disciplined a player, don't hold past misbehavior against that player. Also, never discipline a player for making an error, and don't use physical activity—such as running or doing pushups—as a form of punishment. That sends the message that physical activity is bad.

You shouldn't have to discipline your players too much—especially if you keep them engaged in fun activities throughout practice.

12. Wrap Up the Practice

Sixty minutes flies by, and most coaches want to squeeze as much practice as possible out of their time with their players. But it's helpful to take at least a few minutes to wrap up the practice with a brief meeting.

At this meeting, go over what went well, encourage your players (or have them encourage each other, using the buddy system as described earlier), talk about a few things they still need to work on or give constructive feedback based on what you observed in practice, and remind them of the next game or practice. Send the players off with an encouraging word and a smile.

And make sure you're the last to leave the practice field, so that you know every player got a ride home.

Then, go home yourself—and plan for your next great practice!

THE ABSOLUTE MINIMUM

This chapter was devoted to helping you construct season and practice plans and to knowing how to run effective practices. Among the key points were

- Make a season plan before your season begins so you can see the big picture of what you want to accomplish and plan to teach the skills and tactics in a logical order.

- Be willing to adjust your season plan as necessary, based on what your players need.

- Create a practice plan for each practice, one with a specific purpose. Don't forget to teach rules that are related to the skills and tactics you present in that practice.

- At your first practice, let your players know your goals for the season, your expectations of them, what they can expect from you, what the team rules are (as well as the consequences of breaking them), and what the basic practice structure will be.

- Run simultaneous stations in practice so your players are as active as possible. Develop these stations with players' safety in mind.

- Involve parents in running these stations and in other areas where you could use help.

- Focus these stations on fun, game-like drills and activities. Players who learn skills in the context of how they should be executed in games are best prepared to execute those skills properly in real games.

- Provide skill instruction, feedback on performance, and encouragement. Cultivate a team atmosphere that promotes camaraderie.

- Discipline players as necessary, following through in appropriate ways that steer the players toward better behavior.

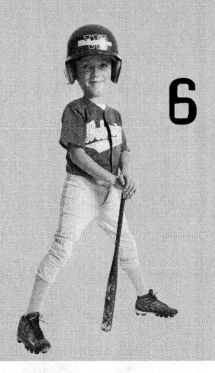

6

PLAYER DEVELOPMENT

Practice time is all about your players learning and developing the skills and tactics they need to successfully execute in games. And that means you have to be a good teacher, a keen observer, a patient guide, and an encouraging critic.

Sound like a lot? It is, but you can learn how to provide this instruction and guidance. And it's critical that you do because, without it, your players will not fully develop their talents and both you and they will be frustrated.

So, get ready to learn how to teach skills and tactics, how to observe your players and give them the feedback they need, and how to correct errors. In Chapter 11, "Games and Drills," you'll find games and drills you can use to teach your players the skills and tactics they need to know.

The Process for Teaching Skills and Tactics

"Hey, this skill is simple. Even I can do it, and I'm not that good. Why can't they do it?"

"I told them how to field ground balls. I was concise, clear, and to the point. Why aren't they doing it right?"

"I spent 10 minutes going into detail on how to field ground balls, but I might as well have been talking to myself, from all the good it did."

Those are among the comments of new coaches, especially if they haven't been in a position to teach before. In the first case, the skill is only simple to the coach, who has likely performed it before. It's not that simple to his players. In the second case, kids need more than an explanation of the skill; they need to see it performed as well. And in the third case, don't mistake the practice field for the lecture hall. Kids don't need a long-winded speech about every minor detail of the skill as it is performed. If you provide one, be prepared for your players to doze off—just as you probably would have at their age.

What *do* your players need? They need you to set the stage for their learning. They need you to show and tell them how to perform the skill or tactic. They need, of course, to practice the skill or tactic. And they need your feedback as they practice.

Set the Stage

The players have just finished warm-ups and Coach Jarvis is ready to practice force outs. He calls the players over to him, but Jake and Deon continue to throw to each other; they don't hear their coach because they're talking as they warm up.

"All right, guys, we're going to have a little infield practice," Coach Jarvis says. Then the coach notices Jake and Deon and calls them over. As they make their way over, Coach Jarvis says, "Let's put an entire infield out there—Matt, Zach, Gary, and Willie—and when you get it, throw to second. All right?"

If Coach Jarvis were a hitter, he would have just struck out. He made three mistakes in setting the stage for this skill instruction:

1. He didn't make sure all his players were listening to him before he began giving instructions.

2. He didn't tell them precisely what they were going to practice.

3. He didn't tell them when or how they would use this skill—whatever it was—in a game.

Why are these things important? Let's look at each issue.

Players' Focus

Coach Jarvis began explaining, in rather cryptic fashion, what the players were going to do before all the players were even within earshot. Even if Coach Jarvis had explained it well, Jake and Deon would have been in the dark about what they were going to be doing.

When you explain a skill or drill to your team, first make sure you have everyone's attention, so practice won't be slowed down as you find yourself explaining things two or three times (see Figure 6.1). Getting your players' attention can sometimes be challenging because two of the main reasons most kids plays sports is they want to have fun and they want to hang out with their friends. Put those two together, and add in other external and internal distractions, and coaches quickly find that they can't assume their players will always be ready to give them their full attention.

> **tip**
>
> To get your players' attention, call them together and make eye contact with each one. If some aren't looking at you, call their names so you make eye contact. Wait until the players are quiet and attentive. If this doesn't happen within a few moments, ask them to stop talking, look at you, and give you their full attention. Don't go on until they do so.

FIGURE 6.1

Get your players' attention before you explain a skill.

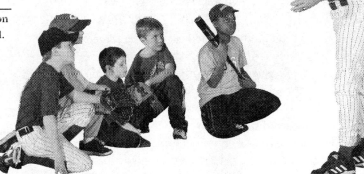

Name That Skill

When you have their attention, identify the skill or tactic you're going to teach. For example, Coach Jarvis should have said something like, "Today we're going to learn how to execute a force out at second base."

Why? For a couple of reasons. First, it gives the players a reference point later. When Coach Jarvis talks about force outs, his players will know what he's referring to. For another, it often helps kids get a mental picture of what they're going to be doing. Mainly, though, it helps avoid confusion later. "Infield practice" covers a wide variety of skills; referring to this won't help your players recall anything. "Force outs at second base" is explicit and clear and will help them recall the skills involved.

Skill Context

During a league game, Jason hits a ball that gets between the outfielders. He rounds first base as the center fielder tries to track the ball down. Jason puts on the brakes and returns to first base, even though he could have easily made it to second without sliding had he continued running.

Between innings, you ask Jason why he didn't continue on to second base. "Because you told us on a hit to the outfield, always round first base," Jason explains.

Never mind that the first base coach should have told Jason to go to second. The real problem is you didn't put the skill of rounding first base into context for Jason. He thought that was just how you ended a hit; he didn't realize you rounded the base, ready to take another base if the play warranted it.

Many coaches do well in getting their players' attention and in naming a skill before they begin to teach it, but they don't realize the importance of putting that skill into context for the players. *You* might understand when a force out situation comes up, how your players should respond, and what will happen if they execute correctly, but your players might not understand these things. And if they don't, chances are they won't successfully execute a force out when the situation arises.

To help them understand, you could ask a few questions such as, "Who can tell me what a force out is?"; "When is a runner forced to run to the next base?"; "What should an infielder try to do if she fields a ground ball in a force out situation?" If you receive a correct answer, make sure everyone heard it and understands it before moving on. If you're not sure whether everyone heard or understands, or if no one gave a correct answer, give a brief, clear answer yourself—something like, "A force-out situation happens when a baserunner is forced to run to the next base on a ground ball, such as when a runner is on first base. On a ground ball when we're on defense, we want to get the force out

note

One of the joys of coaching is when you see your players respond correctly in a situation without telling them what to do. When you put tactics and skills in context of how they're used in a game, your players will learn not just the tactic or skill, but the game itself.

at second if at all possible, so the runner doesn't advance. If an infielder with the ball touches the base before the runner does, the runner is out."

Don't take long with this explanation, but do be clear about when the skill comes up and what its tactical importance is to the team. Let your players know how the team benefits when the skill or tactic is correctly executed.

Show and Tell

Naming the skill and putting it in context should take just a few moments. The next step, "show and tell," will take a little longer.

Some inexperienced coaches make the mistake of *telling* their players how to perform a skill but not *showing* them how. A verbal explanation isn't enough. Neither is just a visual demonstration. If you briefly explain the skill as you demonstrate it, it should sink in (see Figure 6.2).

For example, in teaching how to field a ground ball, you should tell your players how to get in the ready

FIGURE 6.2
Explain the skill as you demonstrate it.

position, move to the ball, and field it, while you are showing them how to do everything you said. The visual demonstration is vital to their comprehension.

Here are a few pointers on what to say about a skill and how to demonstrate it.

What to say:

- Briefly and clearly explain the technique. You should be able to explain the technique for most skills in no more than a minute or two.
- Use language your players understand.
- Ask your players how they are going to perform the skill after you're finished explaining and demonstrating it, to see if they understand what to do.

tip

Watch for comprehension on your players' faces as you explain a skill. If you see a confused look, clear up the confusion before you have the players practice the skill.

What to show:

- Perform the skill as you talk your way through it.
- Show the skill a few times.
- If necessary, use an assistant coach, a parent, or a player to help you demonstrate a skill. You might need to use someone else either to show correct form or to show how two players execute a tactic.
- Break a skill down in parts, showing each part first and then showing the complete skill without a break. For example, on fielding a ground ball, show the ready position. Then show how you move your feet to get in front of a ground ball. Then show how you position your glove and how you watch the ball in your glove. Then show the complete skill all at once.

Practice the Skill

After you've introduced a skill and shown and told your players how to perform it, have them practice the skill in game-like situations. Use drills or games that simulate the experiences they will have in real games and observe their techniques.

Here are suggestions for constructing games and drills that simulate real-game situations and maximize player participation:

- Construct most games with the simultaneous-station idea in mind. That means you'll generally have about five players per game or drill. This allows more opportunities for each player to practice the skill.
- You can also inject some controlled scrimmages during the latter part of the practice, in which you set up plays and have each team execute the plays, keeping score based on their successful executions.
- Focus the action on the skill you want your players to practice, with as little other action surrounding that skill execution as possible. Take care, though, to keep the action realistic, not cutting off too much. In most cases this means making one complete play, beginning with a batted ball and ending with the completion of the play.
- As noted in Chapter 5, "Practice Plans," you should make the games and drills fun. Score them in some way, make them competitive, or add a twist to them while maintaining their realism.
- Construct each game around a singular, clear purpose. Directly tie in to the purpose the successful execution of the skill or tactic.
- Consider ways to make the games a little easier for less talented players and a little harder for more skilled players.

■ Make the games simple to explain and understand. You don't want to spend 5 minutes explaining the game and spend additional time re-explaining it as the players play.

Be sure to see the sample games and drills in Chapter 11 for pitcher, catcher, infielder, outfielder, hitter, baserunner, and offensive and defensive tactics games and drills.

Provide Feedback

As players take part in a drill or game, practicing the skill or tactic you've just taught them, observe their execution and be ready to provide feedback to help them correct errors and improve their play. In this section, you learn about feedback content, timing, whether you should alter your feedback for athletes of varying abilities, and what to do for the kids who just don't seem to get it.

Feedback Content

Focus most of your feedback on the players' attempts to execute the skill you just taught. Don't overload them with feedback as they practice, but do give your hitters coaching cues, such as, "Hands back!" or "Bend your knees!" Similar cues to your fielders might be, "Move your feet!"; "Get in front of it!"; or "Keep your glove down!" These comments are short enough not to distract them and should serve as reminders of the technique you just taught.

However, that doesn't mean you can't provide some feedback concerning related skills. Maybe you just taught the technique for fielding ground balls and now you're conducting a drill or game that calls for infielders to field grounders and make throws to the appropriate base. If fielders are having trouble making accurate throws, you can provide the same type of coaching cues to remind them of proper throwing technique: "Step toward your target!"; "Watch your lead shoulder!"; "Follow through!"

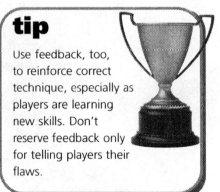

tip

Use feedback, too, to reinforce correct technique, especially as players are learning new skills. Don't reserve feedback only for telling players their flaws.

Feedback Timing

In most cases, the best time to give feedback is as soon as you see something you should comment on, either affirming correct technique or helping a player improve incorrect technique. Many times, as mentioned, you can use coaching cues to remind players of correct technique; you can give these cues as they are participating in the drill or game without stopping the flow.

You can also provide feedback at the end of the drill or game, or at the end of practice, especially if what you have to say applies to multiple players.

If you have feedback that really applies only to one player, in addition to giving feedback on the spot, you can also draw that player aside after the drill or at the end of practice and give him your feedback.

If several of your players are having difficulty performing the skill you just taught and they appear not to know how to go about it, you need to stop the action and reteach the skill. There was a disconnection between your teaching and their learning, and you need to teach the skill in a way that is clear to them—or ask yourself if the skill is too advanced for their ability level. If that's the case, perhaps you need to keep your players focused on refining the fundamental skills.

Altering Your Feedback

Theo, Albert, and Chris are among your players who play in the middle infield.

Theo is a natural in the field. He moves well, covers a lot of ground, has soft hands, can make backhanded plays, and has a good and accurate arm. Theo is a sharp kid, a "quiet leader" type who's always focused and tough internally. He doesn't like to make errors, of course, but he shakes them off when he does.

Albert has some talent, but he is a year younger than Theo, is less mature, and is inconsistent with his mechanics. He appears lackadaisical at times, half-heartedly going after some balls he might have reached with full effort.

Chris has limited range and talent, but he loves the game, tries hard, and gets down on himself when he makes errors or doesn't make plays he thinks he should have. Chris is the least-skilled of the three, though he's more consistent than Albert.

Do you provide the same type of feedback to Theo and Albert? Let's say that on the exact same type of ground ball in the hole, your three fielders do this:

- Theo ranges to his right, makes the backhanded pickup, and fires to first to get the out.
- Albert slows down when he feels he can't reach the ball. You feel, given his range and ability, he could have reached it and gave up on it unnecessarily. Albert shrugs and trots back to his position.
- Chris goes as hard as he can, but the ball just eludes him. Chris shakes his head, upset with himself that he didn't flag down the ball.

With Theo, you tell him, "Way to go!" But what about Albert and Chris? They had the same outcome—they failed to make the play—but you feel Albert could have made the play and gave up on it, while Chris tried his hardest and just couldn't come up with it.

You should applaud Chris for his efforts and encourage him, and you should exhort Albert to go after the ball, while not shaming him in front of his teammates.

The point is that you will be giving feedback on effort and mental approach as well as physical technique. You will be giving feedback to players with a lot of talent, players who have minimal talent, and players who vary in their desires for the game and their emotional makeup.

Shape your feedback to best help the player improve his or her abilities to play the game. Don't panic; this doesn't mean you have to have a different approach for every player. It just means you need to consider what type of feedback will best help the player improve.

Theo and Chris likely won't need any encouragement from you to give it their all. They *will* likely need feedback on technique, but you shouldn't expect Chris to perform at the same level as Theo, so your feedback will be tempered by that and by your understanding that he's hard on himself. You want to focus your feedback on the technical aspects of fielding and give all your players—especially those who, like Chris, are hard on themselves—plenty of encouragement.

As you get to know your players, this tailoring of feedback becomes relatively simple. For now, be aware that, just as your players are individuals, you should shape your feedback according to their individual needs, all with the same end goal in mind: to help them improve their skills.

If at First a Player Doesn't Succeed...

...*don't* ask her to just "try, try again," even though that's how the saying goes. Instead, ask yourself why the player is failing.

Why ask this question? Because a player can make an error for many reasons, and the reason should affect how you respond. Here are some of the reasons:

- The player doesn't know the correct technique.
- She knows the correct technique but doesn't understand the rules or the specific strategy called for.
- She doesn't appear to be giving her full effort.
- She is too anxious about her performance.

Let's consider how you should respond in each situation.

If a player is making errors because she doesn't know the correct technique, she doesn't need your encouragement; she needs your instruction on the mechanics of the skill.

If a player knows the correct technique but makes an error because she's not sure what to do, you need to clarify the rules or explain the strategy called for in that situation.

If a player makes an error or doesn't make a play because of a lack of desire or effort, you need to talk privately with the player and find out why she is giving less than full effort. You should work with the player to eradicate the problem and encourage her to give full effort at all times, both for herself and for her teammates.

If a player is making errors because she is overanxious about her performance, you should talk with this player privately and help her put her performance in perspective. If the anxiety continues, consider moving her to a different spot in the batting order or a different position in the field, with the intent of taking pressure off of her. Help her focus on the technical, physical aspects of the game.

What if a player knows the correct technique, knows the rules and strategies involved, is giving full effort, and isn't overly anxious about her performance but she still makes lots of mistakes?

This youngster needs two things: practice and encouragement. Provide all the opportunities you can for her in practice, and suggest to her parents that they might work with her at home on her skills.

Six Keys to Error Correction

You've heard the saying, "Practice makes perfect." Well, if practice made perfect, then major leaguers would never commit an error. And while practice certainly helps players improve, you will have plenty of technical flaws and other types of errors to correct. Here are six keys to correcting errors:

1. Be encouraging.
2. Be honest.
3. Be specific.
4. Reinforce correct technique.
5. Explain why the error happened.
6. Watch for comprehension.

Let's consider each key.

Be Encouraging

Players are usually discouraged when they commit an error. They need to be corrected, but they also need to be encouraged.

Look for something you can praise, even as you prepare to correct the player. Commend him for his effort. Acknowledge something that he did correctly: "That's the way to get in front of the ball, John." And after you have corrected his technique, end with a smile and a word of encouragement.

Be Honest

Be encouraging, yes, but don't be dishonest. Don't say, "Nice swing, Nick!" if Nick's swing leaves much to be desired. False praise isn't going to help Nick; honesty and correction are.

And don't falsely praise some inconsequential thing, just to give some praise. Kids see through that, and if they know you're not leveling with them, they will be insulted and might question more legitimate comments you make. For exam-

caution

Kids want, and deserve, honesty from you. Otherwise, they'll have to always filter your comments, wondering, "Did he really mean that?"

ple, suppose an infielder throws the ball five feet over the first baseman's head and you, in trying to say something positive, blurt out, "Way to zing the ball over there!" The player will either think you're making fun of him or know you're reaching for a compliment because he threw the ball poorly. Even if he threw it fast, the result was an error, and nothing about the throw could be realistically complimented. You *could*, however, compliment the player for his footwork or his glove work and then tell him how to correct his throwing.

Be Specific

When you correct faulty technique, be specific. During batting practice, don't say, "Come on, Andi! We need you to take better cuts than that!" That doesn't help Andi know what she's doing incorrectly. Rather, say, "Andi, you're wrapping your bat too far behind your head. Hold it at a 45° angle. You can do it."

Focus your correction on the technical aspects the player needs to change, being clear and specific in your comments. Keep your feedback short and precise, and remember to demonstrate the correct action to reinforce your verbal message (see Figure 6.3).

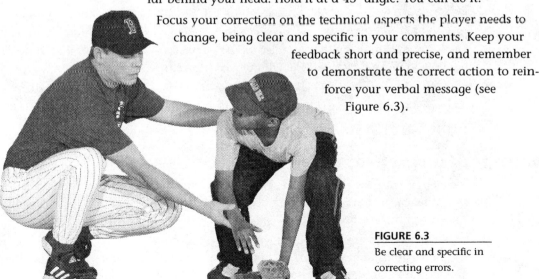

FIGURE 6.3

Be clear and specific in correcting errors.

Reinforce Correct Technique

Ben camps under a fly ball in the outfield and then at the last moment stabs at it with one hand. The ball falls a couple of feet to his side.

Some inexperienced coaches would take the pains to show Ben just what he did wrong: He didn't get under the ball, and he didn't use two hands. And they would be wasting their time.

Why? Because Ben already knows he used incorrect technique. You don't need to demonstrate what he did wrong; he already attempted the catch that way. He needs to see what he *should* do.

Many times, even if you say, "Don't do it this way," or "Here's what you did wrong," as you show the incorrect technique, the player does not hear the message or the incorrect technique is reinforced in his mind's eye because he's seeing it all over again.

Simply show him how to correctly perform the technique, tell him what to do, and let him try it again.

Explain Why the Error Happened

Sometimes kids don't understand what they're doing wrong. You can briefly explain it, without demonstrating the incorrect technique. This explanation can help them understand what they're doing wrong and, as you tell and show them how to execute the skill correctly, they are more likely to get it if they understand what to change.

For example, if an outfielder is crossing her feet as she's tracking a fly ball hit to her side, tell her that that's the reason she wasn't able to cover as much ground as she needed to or that's why she stumbled as she pursued the ball. Then tell and show her how to move in the outfield without crossing your feet.

Most often, however, your players will not need much of an explanation for why they committed the error. Focus most of your time on explaining and demonstrating correct technique.

Watch for Comprehension

Earlier you read about the need to watch for comprehension on your players' faces as you teach them a new skill. You need to watch for this same comprehension as you correct their technique, too.

Look for understanding in your players' eyes and if there's any doubt, ask them, "Do you understand what I mean?" If they don't, couch your verbal message differently, making sure your demonstration of the technique is clear as well.

The effectiveness of your correction is not based on how clear your message is to you; it's based on how well it's received by your players.

THE ABSOLUTE MINIMUM

This chapter focused on your approach to teaching skills and tactics and correcting errors. Key points to remember include

- Remember the method to teaching skills: Set the stage for your players' learning; use a show-and-tell approach to teaching; practice the skill; and provide feedback.

- In setting the stage, make sure your players are listening, name the skill, and put it in context for your players so they can see how they will use it in a game and how correct execution of the skill will benefit the team.

- In the show-and-tell phase, briefly and clearly explain and demonstrate the skill. Watch for player comprehension as you do this, and be ready to clear up any confusion.

- Break down a skill in parts, showing each individual part alone, and then perform the entire skill at once.

- Provide clear feedback to help players improve their skills.

- Consider reasons why players are making errors and tailor your feedback accordingly. Sometimes they might not know how to perform the skill and need skill instruction; at other times they might understand how to perform the skill but need help improving their mechanics. They also might not understand the rules or strategies that relate to the situation.

- When correcting errors, keep these six keys in mind: Be encouraging; be honest; be specific; reinforce correct technique; explain why the error happened; and watch for comprehension.

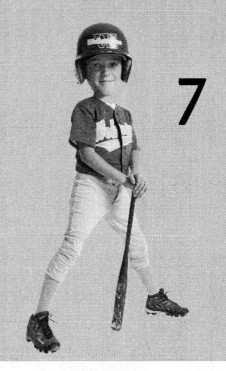

7

GAME TIME!

The bleachers begin to fill with parents, grandparents, and siblings of players. The players arrive singly and in pairs, looking crisp and sharp in their uniforms. The foul lines are chalked, the umpires are on hand, and the field is freshly mown and green. As your players warm up, you can see the excitement in their faces.

A few butterflies stir to life in your stomach. For every butterfly fluttering in your stomach, you figure there must be a dozen in your players' bellies. Anticipation, hope, anxiety, and joy intermingle in the air. In a few minutes, the home plate umpire will yell those magical words, "Play ball!"; the first batter will stride to the plate, bat in hand; and the game will begin.

There's nothing like game time, nothing like that first pitch of the game, winging home like an airborne messenger, releasing the tension that had been building since the first players arrived for warm-ups.

Playing games is really what it's all about. Kids come to practice to learn and hone skills with one purpose in mind: to play as well as possible during games. It takes planning and expertise to make practices fun, but playing league games is *inherently* fun, and the main reason that most kids sign up for baseball.

So far, you've learned to apply the keys to coaching to your practices. In this chapter you learn to apply those keys before, during, and after games. What should you communicate to your players at the practice before a game? When the game rolls around, do you change your approach to coaching in any way? How should you construct your lineup and rotate players in and out? How much teaching and error correction should you do during a game? How much strategy should you employ during a game? What should you tell players before and after a game? For the answers to these and many similar questions, read on.

The Practice Before the Game

For the most part, the practice immediately preceding a game will not differ from any other practice. But there are a few things you need to discuss with your players, including the game particulars and the team's tactical focus for the game.

Game Particulars

At the end of the practice, remind the players of the game time, the field location, and what time you want them to arrive at the field to warm up. Tell them to arrive 20 minutes before the game so they have enough time to warm up—and so you can see who is there and make out your lineup card. Remind them to wear their team uniforms and bring their gloves.

Many games are played around dinnertime or shortly after. Give your players some guidance on what to eat, what not to eat, and how soon before a game they should eat. See the following sidebar, "Fueling Up," for guidelines on what players should eat and drink before, during, and after games.

FUELING UP

It's 20 minutes before game time. Do you know what's in your players' stomachs? Whatever it is, they will use it as the fuel in their tanks for the game.

Hopefully, their fuel doesn't consist of a big steak dinner or a couple of fast-food burgers lathered in "special" (read: fat-laden) sauce, with a large order of fries, washed down with a soft drink.

Why? Because foods high in fat take longer to digest. Your players should have easily digested food in their stomachs, so their energy goes toward playing rather than digesting.

The carbonation in soft drinks can cause indigestion, and the sugar content results in a rise in blood insulin levels, which can make players tired. Tell your players not to have soft drinks within a few hours of a game.

That doesn't mean they should show up empty-stomached. That's like taking off on a drive with your gas tank all but dry.

Players should have something light and digestible an hour or two before the game—a bagel or toast and a little fruit would be good, though a lot of fruit can cause gastrointestinal stress. Some cereal to tide them over until after the game works, too.

> **tip**
> If a game is canceled, a phone tree is a great way to get the word out quickly while not taking a lot of your own time. Just set up a system so you're sure that everyone is called.

If they have time, they can eat a light meal two to three hours before the game. This meal should be high in carbohydrates and low in fat.

As for fluids, players should drink water before, during, and after a game. Sports drinks are good, too, and provide the added benefit of replacing minerals and electrolytes lost through exercise and sweat. Players should drink two or three cups of water or sports drink (24–30 ounces) within two hours of a game and drink about 8 ounces of fluid every 20 minutes during a game.

Game Focus

Your team's tactical focus might consist solely of executing the fundamentals well—and if your team does that, it has an excellent chance of winning. Especially at younger levels of play, there isn't much need for intricate tactics; you want your players to simply focus on executing the individual skills well.

At the younger levels, your strategy should be easily remembered, with much or all of it becoming part of your season-long mantra: "Swing at good pitches. Keep your eye on the ball. Watch the ball in your glove. Know what you're going to do with the ball. Be aggressive."

> **tip**
> Don't just dictate team strategy for older players; ask their input. This helps them to consider their strengths and the strategies that would help them win. It also results in them perhaps more fully buying into the strategies because they had a part in designing them.

If you are coaching older or more experienced players, however, you can and should consider your tactical approach to the game. This approach hinges on your players' strengths and abilities and on the opponent you're facing.

What are some of the team tactical approaches you might consider?

- **Use your team speed to manufacture runs**—This is always good to do and is especially useful when facing a tough pitcher.

- **Move runners over**—Look to use the sacrifice bunt, the hit-and-run, and hitting to the right side to move runners into scoring position.

- **Rattle the pitcher**—Sometimes a pitcher's concentration can be broken, and his effectiveness diminished, by baserunners who can rattle him by bluffing steals or stealing bases. When baserunners can attract as much attention as the batter, the pitcher is in trouble.

- **Make the pitcher throw strikes**—Many times batters help pitchers by swinging at balls out of the strike zone. When a team is focused and disciplined at the plate, good things happen. They get walks; they force the pitcher to throw the ball down the center of the plate to get strikes because it's hard for young pitchers to nibble at the corners of the plate; and they swing at pitches that are hitters' pitches, thus generally hitting the ball harder. In addition, a pitcher might tire more quickly because he has thrown more pitches. This is a good tactic especially if the pitcher is talented but a little wild. Forcing him to throw more pitches increases the chances that he will have to come out of the game at some point.

Individual tactics and strategies you can employ during a game include

- **Stolen bases, including double steals**—A double steal generally happens when runners on first and second steal on the same play.

- **Squeeze bunts, including safety squeezes and suicide squeezes**—A *safety squeeze*, you'll recall from Chapter 2, "Rules of the Game," occurs when a batter bunts with a runner on third base and the runner breaks for home as soon as the bunt is on the ground. A *suicide squeeze* begins the same way, but the runner on third breaks for home as soon as the rules allow before the batter has made contact, thus either scoring easily if the batter gets the ball on the ground or being put out easily at the plate if the batter misses the ball.

- **Hit-and-run plays**—A *hit-and-run* occurs with at least one runner on base and moving on the pitch as the batter tries to put the ball into play. These are best employed with a batter who has a good chance of hitting the ball.

- **Playing the infield in to cut off the runner headed home from third base**—With a drawn-in infield, it's much harder for the runner to score if an infielder fields the ball, but it's also easier for a ground ball to get through the infield, so it's a calculated risk.

- **Double plays**—Double plays can be made in a number of ways: a strike 'em out, throw 'em out in which a batter strikes out and the catcher throws out a would-be base-stealer, a line drive caught by an infielder who doubles a runner off a base, and a fly ball caught by an outfielder who throws out a baserunner trying to advance after tagging up are three examples. One of the more common examples of a double play at upper levels of play (but difficult to pull off at lower levels) is the ground ball double play—for example, a 6-4-3, in which a shortstop fields a grounder and tosses it to the second baseman to force the runner on first and the second baseman fires to first to beat the batter/runner as well. Ground ball double plays require sure hands, quick feet, and strong accurate arms.

Before the Game

Arrive about 30 minutes before game time, if possible. Use the 10 minutes or so that you have before your players arrive to check the field. Just as you do before practices, look for broken glass, potholes, or any other hazards and take care of them if you can. If you can't, talk with the opposing coach and umpires about how to ensure players' safety, and report the problem to your league administrator after the game.

In addition to checking the field, you have three other duties to tend to before the game begins: making sure your team warms up properly, filling out your lineup card, and giving your players a few pearls of wisdom before they take to the field.

Team Warm-up

This is simple enough, and players should know the routine from practice. They need to jog a few minutes, stretch, and throw to loosen up their arms. In addition, the starting pitcher and catcher should warm up together, with the catcher receiving pitches in the normal catching position, with the catcher's equipment on. You or an assistant coach should supervise the pitcher/catcher warm-up as well as the entire team's warm-up.

Lineups

Lineups can be tricky to concoct if players show up just a few minutes before game time, or not at all; if you've made out your lineup card at home, just be ready to change it at the last minute.

If you plan to play everyone an equal amount of time, as is often the case at younger levels of competition, there's not a tremendous amount of difference in making out the lineup card; you just have to figure out how to get everyone in. This issue is addressed later in this chapter. At older levels, as you play your better players more, some strategy does come into play in making out your lineup. Here are some of the desired attributes and characteristics of the hitters in a batting order:

#1 (The leadoff hitter) Good eye, good speed, contact hitter, good on-base percentage, and good baserunner.

#2 Good bat control, ability to hit to all fields (including right field, to move the runner over), good contact hitter (for hit-and-run plays), and good on-base percentage.

#3 Often the best hitter on the team. Hits for power and for average.

#4 (Cleanup hitter) Often the biggest slugger on the team. Hits for power and for average.

#5 Another power hitter.

#6 Hits for less power than #s 3–5, but has better bat control and doesn't strike out as much. Good line drive hitter.

#7 Similar to #2 hitter, with perhaps more extra-base ability, but probably doesn't hit for as high an average or get on base as often.

#8 One of your weaker hitters.

#9 Probably your weakest hitter.

> **note**
>
> One coach I know kept the same batting order throughout the entire season and began the next game with the batter who was due up next when the final out was made. Most of the players got to lead off a game at one time or another. This is especially useful for younger kids because they get accustomed to knowing who they follow and everyone gets a chance to lead off, but it's not recommended for older, more competitive levels of play.

In terms of defense, desired attributes were covered in the section "Players" in Chapter 2.

In "Player Substitutions" later in this chapter, you'll consider options in rotating players in and out of the lineup, in rotating players at various positions, and in playing time issues.

Last-minute Words

As noted in Chapter 3, "Communication Keys," you don't need to fire up your troops with a dramatic pep talk. But you do need to help them prepare to compete, and a few well-chosen words before the game can do just that.

Remind them to focus on the basics and to execute the fundamental skills and tactics they have been practicing. Go over any particular strategies or game plans you discussed in the previous practice. You might also note how you will substitute players in, although you don't necessarily need to divulge this. Sometimes, however, it's easy enough to let players know the general approach to when and how they will be subbed in, and this can help them get mentally prepared.

Above all, tell them to play hard and have fun.

Your talk might go something like this: "All right, guys, just make the play in front of you—watch the ball into your glove and make good, strong throws. At the plate, be aggressive, but don't swing at bad pitches. Let's look to take the extra base and put the pressure on the defense. Let's play hard, play smart, and have fun. Are you ready?"

This will help focus your players on the fundamentals, remind them of the game plan, and keep the big picture in mind.

During the Game

You know your role as coach at practice and how to plan for practices and run them effectively.

But what, if anything, changes for you during games? Does your coaching role change? Is there a subtle shift in your approach? Do you do the same amount of coaching and the same type of coaching? How do you respond to players' errors, and how do you plan to rotate your players in and out?

This section takes a look at your role as coach during the game, providing strategies and tips to help you effectively guide your players throughout the contest.

Your Approach to the Game

During every practice, your focus is on helping your players acquire and develop the physical skills, tactical abilities, and mental approach and understanding to do what? To compete, with the goal of winning clearly in mind. Winning is the common goal of every team. Your job is to prepare your players in a way that puts them in a position to compete and to win.

Your job is also, as stated in Chapter 1, "Your Coaching Approach," to not over-emphasize winning. Or, more directly put, to emphasize player development over winning. Of course, when you emphasize this development, you increase your chances of winning, so you're not working against yourself or your players here.

This all sounds so much easier than it really is. The pressure to win is enormous, and the inclination among players and coaches alike is to define themselves according to their win-loss record or personal achievements.

If you approach the game in a way that reinforces that winning-is-everything mentality in players' minds, you are doing them a disservice. If your coaching decisions reflect your concern first for your players and their development, and then your desire to win, you have the right approach. But you have to consciously go into each game with this mindset because the common mindset runs contrary to this.

Other considerations in your approach include how much coaching you do, what type of coaching you provide, how you employ strategies in your game plan, and how you address or correct errors during games. Let's examine these issues one at a time.

How Much Coaching?

How much coaching you do during a game depends on what your players need. You don't want to over-coach, and you don't want to under-coach.

Some of the signs of over-coaching include

- You have an intricate set of signals for your hitters and baserunners that most major league players would have difficulty understanding.
- You prepare and rehearse a 5-minute pep talk aimed solely at "firing up" the troops.
- You never stop talking throughout the game. You give each of your hitters a detailed analysis of how to hit, and you give each of your fielders specific instructions before every new batter.
- When a player makes an error, you pull him aside in between innings and give him detailed skill instruction.
- You spend hours analyzing your team's statistics after games.
- You get all over the 16-year-old umpire because you think he missed a borderline pitch.
- You warm up a 9-year-old left-handed relief pitcher in anticipation of facing a left-handed hitter the next inning.
- You send a scout to watch your next opponent's practice.
- You contest a close play at the plate, even though you see that your player was clearly out, in hopes of "softening up" the umpire for other close plays later in the game.

Almost as bad as over-coaching is under-coaching. Some of the signs of under-coaching include

- You don't tell your players what to focus on before the game begins; you simply show up, write out the lineup card, wish your players "Good luck," and settle in to watch the game.

▨ You don't provide any brief coaching tips or cues to your hitters and fielders.

▨ When a player asks you for some specific guidance, you just clap your hands and say, "Do your best."

▨ You give no instructions to your baserunners.

▨ You give no encouragement to your players.

▨ One of your players is losing his cool and is on the borderline of being thrown out of the game, and you don't intervene.

▨ One of your players is upset about an error he has made, and he sits in tears on the bench as you sit, passive and mute, a few feet away.

▨ Your pitcher is very wild or is getting hit hard and is embarrassed about his performance, but you leave him in because you had him scheduled to go four innings.

There are some extreme examples in both of those lists, but they aren't so extreme, unfortunately, as to be rare. What you should aim for is something that falls between over- and under-coaching. What's the right amount of coaching in youth baseball? Here are seven keys to coaching effectively during games:

▨ **Help your players get mentally prepared**—Remind them of their focus for the game and of any game plan that you devised in the previous practice. Keep them zoned in on properly executing the fundamentals. They will have nervous energy; you need to help them direct and expend that energy in ways that will help them compete well.

▨ **Provide tactical direction**—Guide your players in the appropriate tactics as situations arise. Don't expect them to automatically know what to do in each situation. Let them know you want to try to get a double play or want the infield to come in for the play at the plate, or give them a signal for a sacrifice bunt if that's what you want to do.

▨ **Be involved, and be encouraging**—Part of being involved happens as you provide that tactical direction. Stay in the game mentally and emotionally. Encourage your players, and foster that same type of support among the players themselves.

▨ **Give technique tips and reminders**—Don't go into full-blown, detailed instruction on skills; save that for the next practice if you see that players are not executing correctly. Giving too much instruction during a game takes a player's focus off the game itself. But *do* give technique tips and reminders, cues that will help them remember what you taught them in practice: "Keep your foot in there! Don't bail out!" "Watch the ball into your glove!" "Nice level swing now!" "Step toward your target!" These technique tips should be enough to remind them of the more complete instruction you gave at previous practices.

- **Let the players play**—Guide your players, yes, but don't be like a puppeteer, with invisible strings attached to them, prompting their every move. It's your duty to teach them the skills and tactics and to let them experience the game as they compete against other teams. You coach and direct during games, but not with such a heavy hand that your players can't, or don't want to, think for themselves. Part of the joy for the players is learning how to perform and make decisions in games. Beyond ensuring that all your players get in the game, don't make numerous personnel moves, and don't constantly shout out instructions. Keep in the game, give players technique tips and encouragement, and let them play.

- **Tend to your players' needs**—Letting your players play doesn't mean you don't tend to their needs. Remind them before the game of your tactical approach or game plan. Give them coaching tips, support, and encouragement. If a player is disconsolate, tend to him; if a player twists an ankle, tend to her. Provide general direction throughout the game. And supply one more thing, which is the final item in this list.

- **Help your players keep the proper perspective**—Many coaches provide essentially everything their players need, except for this last item: keeping the game in perspective. These coaches build up each game as if it's a World Series encounter and celebrate wins excessively while moping or grousing about the umpires in defeat. Their players, of course, tend to take their cues from these coaches. The players make more of victories than they should, and they are poor sports or depressed in defeat, sulking or obsessing over a play they could have made that might have turned the game around.

Don't do this to your players! Don't make more of a victory than it is because then kids get too wrapped up in the game's outcome, which they can't control. Keep them focused on their performances, which they *can* control. Even in victory, there are things to improve, and even in defeat, there are successes to be found. Help your players enjoy the game, to play it hard and as well as they can, and to learn from both wins and losses, while keeping both in proper perspective. It is, after all, a game. And it should be left on the field, win or lose. Young hearts and minds shouldn't labor long over a loss, and young heads shouldn't become so large after a win that players have difficulty pulling their shirts off when they get home.

Positive Coaching

Imagine Coach Swanson, in irritation or anger, shouting these comments during a game, for everyone (his players, opposing players, and fans) to hear:

"Come on, Nathan! How many times have I told you to stay down on ground balls!"

"Lucas! What kind of swing is that? You are *not* doing what I told you to do!"

"Ann, you have to charge that ball! You let a run score by waiting for it to come to you!"

Chances are pretty good that Nathan, Lucas, and Ann will play the rest of the game with one eye on their coach, hoping not to make another play that draws Coach Swanson's ire or derogatory comments. Nathan and Ann probably will be happy if no more balls are hit their way, and Lucas probably won't mind if he doesn't get to hit again.

There's something about public humiliation that makes kids tentative.

Yet way too many coaches publicly humiliate their players, either consciously or unconsciously. These are the same coaches who attach too much importance to winning, who conveniently forget to put in their least-skilled players (or try to hide them in the field for half an inning), and who grouse all game long at the umpires.

It would have been far more appropriate if Coach Swanson had taken Nathan, Lucas, and Ann aside—not in a huge public display, but privately—and calmly given each child the brief technique tip that he or she needed, along with an encouraging pat on the back before sending him or her back out on the field.

Look to build up your players, not tear them down. Teach in a positive manner, and keep control of your own emotions. Keep your comments focused on the techniques players need to improve, delivering them in a way that lets players know you are on their side. Remind them of times in the past when they performed the skill well. Help them to see themselves successfully performing it, and show by your words and body language that you believe they can do it again.

caution

Remember, if your body language belies your words—if you say, "You can do it," but your shoulders are sagging and you look irritated or disbelieving—the player will not believe your positive words.

Appropriate Strategy

Again, at the younger levels, your main strategy is to have your players execute the fundamentals. As the players gain in age, size, experience, and ability, you can begin to employ various strategies to help your team win. And, as noted earlier, when you involve your players in some of these strategy decisions and they have input into the game plan, they enjoy the game more, develop their ability to understand the mental and tactical aspects of the game, and feel more of a buy-in to the plan. It therefore helps them develop as players.

Put your players in situations where they are most likely to succeed and where they are most talented. If your players are not fleet of foot and you're going up against the league's best catcher in terms of throwing out base stealers, it's obviously not wise to employ a running game. If you want to hit-and-run but your batter is one who swings and misses more often than not and your runner on first base is slow, you should rethink your strategy. Keep your strategy in line with your players' skill levels and the game situation.

Minimal Error Correction

Your players are going to commit errors. In most cases, you'll have multiple errors in a game that you will need to address. So much of coaching is helping players correct errors. So, how should you approach this duty during games?

First, note the types of errors that are made by more than one player. You should address the necessary skill execution for the entire team in your next practice.

Second, note errors made by individual players. Perhaps Bobby has a tendency to try to catch fly balls with one hand and drops more than he catches. Or maybe Matt doesn't move his feet well enough to get in front of ground balls and makes errors on his backhanded attempts more often than not. Give Bobby and Matt brief instruction during the game, reminding them of the proper techniques they have been taught.

Games are for playing, not for detailed instruction. Your players' focus should be on the game. Save the more detailed instruction and technique practice for your next practice.

Score Sheets

Score sheets are used to keep track of what each batter does in the game. You can use them to keep track of runs and outs in each half inning as well as statistics on your own players. For a sample score sheet, see Figure 7.1.

FIGURE 7.1

Sample score
sheet.

Sample Scorebook

#	Lineup	Pos	1	2	3	4	5	6	7	8	9	10	AB	R	H	RBI

Visitor: / Home: | Start Time: / End Time: | Weather: / Scorer: | Date: / Time of Game:

SUMMARY
Runs / Hits / Errors / Left on Base

#	Opposing Pitchers	W/L/S	IP	H	R	ER	BB	SO	HB	BK	TBF

#	Catchers	PB

Umpires
HP: / 2B:
1B: / 3B:

Keeping score can be as simple or as complex as you make it. There are many differ-ent ways to keep score, but here are some basics:

- Use the player position numbers when noting a fielding play: 1 = pitcher, 2 = catcher, and so on. See the section "Players" in Chapter 2 to refresh your memory of player position numbers, if you need to.

- For each out recorded, write the number of the out (1, 2, or 3) in the lower-right side of the box for the player on whose at-bat the out was recorded. Then circle that out. This helps you to easily track the number of outs each half inning (see Figure 7.2).

FIGURE 7.2
The second out of the inning is recorded.

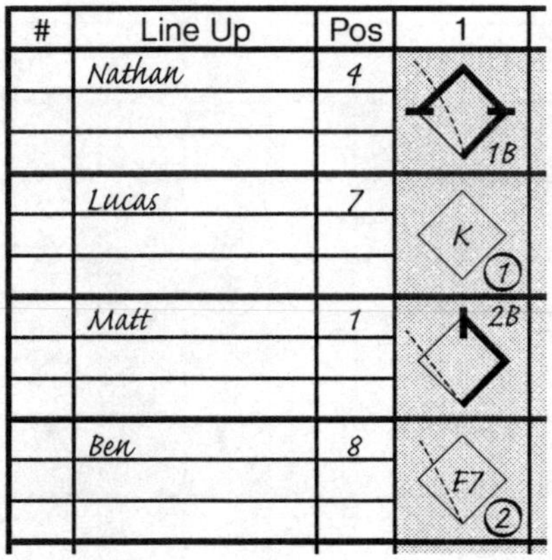

- For each run scored, darken in the diamond for the runner who scored (see Figure 7.3).

FIGURE 7.3
Three runners score on the home run.

■ Record ground-outs by using the player position numbers involved. For example, "6-3" means the batter hit a ground ball to the shortstop (6), who threw the batter out at first base (3). See Figure 7.4.

■ Record fly-outs and pop-outs by noting *F* and the position number of the fielder who caught the ball. For example, "F7" denotes a fly-out to the left fielder, and "F4" means the second baseman caught a pop-up (see Figure 7.5).

■ Record strikeouts by writing a *K* in the box of the batter who struck out. Some coaches write a backwards *K* to indicate a called third strike—in other words, the batter didn't swing and miss; he was called out on strikes (see Figure 7.6). Another way to indicate a called third strike is to write "Kc" (the *c* stands for "called").

■ Record a single, double, triple, or home run by writing "1B," "2B," "3B," or "HR" (see Figure 7.7).

■ Note baserunner progress by marking the baseline up to the base the runner advances to on each individual play. For example, the runner in Figure 7.8 singled, advanced to second on a ground ball, and advanced to third after tagging up on a fly ball but did not score. If he had scored, his diamond would have been darkened in.

FIGURE 7.7

The first four batters hit a single, double, triple, and home run, respectively.

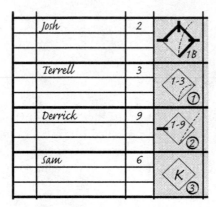

#	Line Up	Pos	1
	Nathan	4	
	Lucas	7	
	Matt	1	
	Ben	8	

FIGURE 7.8

The batter singled, advanced to second base on a ground out, and went to third base on a fly ball.

	Josh	2	
	Terrell	3	
	Derrick	9	
	Sam	6	

- If desired, note the location of the ball (whether it's a hit or an out) with a dotted line, as shown in several of the previous figures.

- Note an error on a fielder by writing *E* and the player's position number. For example, an error by the third basemen is "E5" (see Figure 7.9).

FIGURE 7.9

Error by the third baseman.

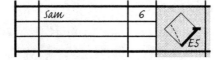

	Sam	6	

For a sample half inning, see Figure 7.10. In it, the first batter singles to left field. He then steals second base. The second batter hits a base hit to center field, scoring the runner on second. The third hitter flies out to left field. The fourth hitter singles to center field, and the runner on first goes to third. The fifth hitter hits a sacrifice fly to right field, scoring the runner on third, while the runner on first base remains at first. The sixth hitter hits a double to left, scoring the runner on first. The seventh hitter strikes out for the third out. Three runs are scored in the half inning.

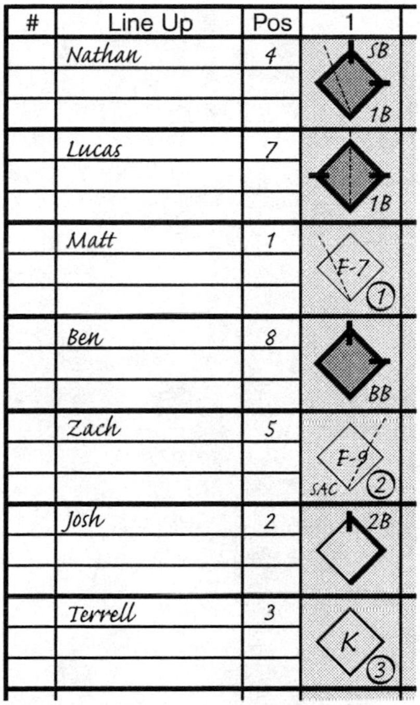

FIGURE 7.10

Sample half inning.

#	Line Up	Pos	1
	Nathan	4	SB / 1B
	Lucas	7	1B
	Matt	1	F-7 ①
	Ben	8	BB
	Zach	5	F-9 SAC ②
	Josh	2	2B
	Terrell	3	K ③

Now for some basic notations to use on your score sheet:

- 1B = single
- 2B = double
- 3B = triple
- BB = base on balls, or walk
- BK = balk
- CS = caught stealing
- DP = double play
- E = error
- FC = fielder's choice (occurs when at least two runners are on base and the fielder makes a choice regarding where to get the out)
- G = ground ball
- HBP = hit by pitcher
- HR = home run

- K = strikeout
- LD = line drive (this augments the basic score keeping, helping you remember the nature of the play)
- PB = passed ball (similar to a wild pitch, but the catcher should have caught the ball; a passed ball allows a runner to advance to the next base)
- RBI = run batted in
- Sac = sacrifice
- SB = stolen base
- WP = wild pitch (similar to a passed ball, but the catcher could not have caught or stopped the ball from getting away and allowing a runner to advance)

tip

To denote one or more runs batted in (RBIs), write "RBI" in the box of the player who drove in the run, along with the number of runs driven in on the play. You can also denote other plays, such as fielder's choice (FC), stolen base (SB), hit by pitch (HBP), line drives (LD), and so on.

There is no one correct way to keep score. If you go online or to a sporting goods store, you'll find various types of scorebooks and score sheets. Find one that works for you before the season begins, consider the best way for you to log the information you want to log, and have fun with it.

Player Substitutions

There are three issues to consider as you plan your player substitutions:

- Playing time
- Rotating players at various positions
- In-game substitutions

Playing Time

Is equal playing time appropriate? Is it fair? Should your less talented players play as much as your more talented players?

The first question to answer is actually this one: Does your league require equal playing time? Some leagues do, but some don't. Often, as the kids get older, this requirement—if in place at all—is dropped.

If it is in place, you need to have a plan that results in your players getting the same number of innings.

If it's not in place, you need to decide whether you think an equal-playing-time policy is fitting. There are two camps of thought here. They go something like this:

- **For equal playing time**—"The outcome of the game isn't as important as it is for the players to develop their skills and have fun. How are the lesser-skilled players going to develop their skills if they don't play? And what's the fun of sitting on the bench?"

- **Against equal playing time**—"Why punish the better players by sitting them down, and why risk losing by playing your lesser-skilled players as much as your more talented athletes? That's not teaching the kids realistic lessons about competition, anyway, because in all other aspects of life the emphasis is on winning and the attitude is dog-eat-dog."

Equal playing time makes sense, whether it's league policy or not, for players eight years old and younger. After that, playing time should shift more and more to the better players, though lesser-skilled players should still get decent chunks of playing time at ages 9 and 10. By 11 and 12, most of the playing time normally goes to the better athletes.

So, let's say you plan to give your players equal playing time, and you have 13 players show up for a six-inning game. How do you evenly divide the playing time?

One way you could figure it is this:

- Multiply the number of position players on the field by the number of innings played: 9 positions × 6 innings = 54. In other words, there are 54 position slots during a 6-inning game with 9 fielders.

- Take this figure and divide by the number of players who showed up: 54 slots divided by 13 players = 4.15. That's the number of innings each player should get. Obviously, you can't play 4.15 innings, but all players should play at least 4 full innings, and a few will play 5.

So, how would that play out? In Figure 7.11, the 13 players are labeled Players A–M. Let's say Players A–C are your three best players; these players are shaded dark. Players D–J are average players; these players are shaded medium. Players K–M are lesser-skilled players; these players are not shaded. Let's further assume your league's substitution rule is a player can reenter a game once after being subbed for.

Based on the sample shown in Figure 7.11, here's how it breaks down:

- Your top two players get five innings, while everyone else gets four.

- Your three least-skilled players play four innings apiece but don't play in the final inning. However, they get their fair share.

- Seven of your nine players in innings 1, 2, and 5 are among your stronger players.
- All nine players in the final inning are among your stronger players.

FIGURE 7.11

Player substitution sample.

Player	Inning						
	1	2	3	4	5	6	Total Innings
A	X	X	X		X	X	5
B	X	X	X		X	X	5
C	X	X	X			X	4
D	X	X		X	X		4
E	X	X	X			X	4
F	X			X	X	X	4
G	X			X	X	X	4
H			X	X	X	X	4
I		X		X	X	X	4
J		X	X	X		X	4
K	X		X	X	X		4
L	X	X	X	X			4
M		X	X	X	X		4
Players on Field	9	9	9	9	9	9	

The main point here is to think out your plan before you get to the field. You might want to work out, before your season begins, three separate substitution plans, based on different numbers of players showing up. For example, if you are assigned 15 players, make out substitution samples as shown in Figure 7.11 for 13, 14, and 15 players showing up. Bring each sample to the field with you, and then use whichever one applies for that game.

Rotating Players in Different Positions

Rotating players in and out of the lineup is one issue; rotating players in different positions is another. The question here is, do you have players specialize at one or two positions, do you give every player relatively equal time in every position, or do you do something in between?

As with the equal playing time issue, there are different schools of thought on this subject. A couple of them go something like this:

- **Don't move players around in different positions**—"If Greg can't field ground balls, why put him at shortstop and make it evident to the whole world? And why embarrass him in doing so? Besides, kids won't develop their fielding skills at any one position if they keep getting bounced around. You're harming the players by doing this, not helping them."

▓ **Give players equal playing time at all positions**—"Youth baseball is all about learning the various positions and getting a feel for each one. Later kids can begin to specialize. Besides, the shifting around emphasizes the fact that, at this level, the game's focus is on learning, player development, and fun."

There is truth to each school of thought. Consider the following guidelines as you decide whether to rotate players and, if so, how often you should rotate them and to how many positions.

Players 6–8 Years Old

For ages 6–8, rotate players freely in coach-pitch or machine-pitch situations. This is their introduction to the sport, and there's no reason to pigeonhole kids at this point.

However, use some discretion in rotating. If you have a child who is absolutely terrified of catching throws, don't put him at first base until he becomes comfortable catching thrown balls.

Also, if players are pitching at any of these ages, don't rotate all players through the positions of pitcher and catcher. Choose pitchers who can get the ball over the plate (no, there's no painting the corners of the plate at these ages, unless it happens by accident!), and select catchers who want to be behind the plate and who can catch well.

When you rotate, choose one option or the other: either inning by inning, or game by game. I've seen both situations work well, though I would use the inning-by-inning approach only for younger players and have a set strategy for player rotation there, as opposed to making it up on-the-fly every inning. For example, every player could simply move down one position number in the order each inning—the second baseman (4) in the third inning becomes the third baseman (5) in the fourth, while the third baseman moves to shortstop (6), and so on. Admittedly, it's easier rotating game by game.

Players 9+ Years Old

If you are coaching 9-year-olds or above, you might still rotate players some, but be more selective about your rotation, and it's good to settle on one or two positions for most players at this point. Why? They've had the opportunity to play in most or all of the positions, and it's time for them to begin to develop the skills that are specific to one or two positions.

Generally, group your players by areas: pitchers and catchers (and you probably will have two catchers, one being a backup who plays elsewhere and only catches when the starting catcher isn't playing), infielders, and outfielders. You can rotate some among the infielders and outfielders (meaning an infielder might move to another infield position, and an outfielder to another outfield position), but by and large, stick with placing your players in the positions where they will most excel and help the team.

In-game Substitutions

One of your game responsibilities is to make substitutions. At the earlier ages, make your substitutions to ensure all players get about equal playing time; this was already covered in the section "Playing Time." For ages 9 and above, here are some ideas for making substitutions:

- **Pitching changes**—Don't allow your pitcher to throw more than 75 pitches in a game. Change pitchers at or before this point to protect the pitcher's arm. Also, change pitchers if your pitcher is showing signs of wearing down—if she is having trouble finding the strike zone or is being hit hard.

- **Defensive changes**—Put your strongest defense on the field in the last inning or two, if they're not already in place.

- **Pinch-hitting**—Sometimes players are better hitters than they are fielders. As you progress to competitive situations where you play your better players more, you might have one or two pinch-hitting specialists who are great to use in the right late-inning situation.

> **caution**
>
> You need to be aware of your league rules regarding substitutions. Some leagues allow a player who has played and been substituted for to reenter the game once. This rule will affect how you plan for your substitutions.

Appropriate Behavior

Remember that all eyes are upon you, at one time or another, during a game. Of most importance are the eyes of your players. They see how you behave, and that greatly impacts how they behave, or at least how they think they should behave.

Be positive, be encouraging, and cheer your team on. If you want to discuss a play with an umpire, do so respectfully. And in many cases you can do so between innings, unless you need to question a call that might be changed during an inning.

Coach your players to be good sports, and lead the way by being one yourself. Don't argue with opposing coaches, don't say derogatory things to opposing players, and don't root *against* the opposing team. Simply root *for* your team.

Coach your players to play hard, to play fair, and to play to win. Let your players know in advance how you will respond if they do or say something unsporting at a game, and follow through. For a mild infraction of your rules, talk to them, correct them, and give them one more chance. For a second mild infraction, take them out of the game. For a major infraction, even if it's the first, take them out of the game. In either case, consider suspending them for another game if you believe the infraction warrants such a response.

Sports offer an arena for kids to not only practice their physical skills, but also learn discipline, the proper expression of emotion, patience, and respect for themselves and others. And the person they learn most from is you.

After the Game

After the game, line your players up for a team handshake with their opponents. (Instruct your players in practice how you want them to behave during this post-game handshake.) Have them shake or slap hands and offer "Good game" or some similar comment to their opponents. Be clear with your players that you want them to refrain from saying anything derogatory, no matter what happened during the game. The team handshake is an important part of youth sports because it teaches respect for the opponent and helps keep the contest in perspective.

If you win, celebrate, but do so in a manner that doesn't rub it in to the other team. If you lose, don't hang your heads. Either way, go through the team handshake, thank the umpires for taking their time to umpire the game, and then return to your side of the field for a brief post-game meeting.

Team Meeting

Hold a brief meeting before letting the kids go. This isn't the time to go into great detail, but let them know what they did well, what they still need to work on, and give them some positives to take home. Note areas where they have improved, note plays or situations in which they performed well, and help them keep the outcome in perspective. Help them learn from the game, whether they won or lost. For some thoughts on what you can learn from winning and losing, see the following sidebar, "Lessons of the Game."

Finally, remind your players of the next practice or game, and make sure they all have rides before you leave the field. Don't leave a child waiting for a ride, even if he says he's waiting to be picked up by a parent; make sure he gets his ride before you leave.

LESSONS OF THE GAME

What can players learn from a win? They can learn that

- Hard effort sometimes pays off. So, maybe all that time spent in practice is worth it after all!

- Sometimes you're better than the other team, and it shows. But don't rest on your laurels because another game is coming.

- Sometimes you get lucky. The best team doesn't always win, and your team can win on any given day.

- Winning is a team effort. Contributions to a win can come from unexpected places.

A win feels great, so celebrate. But remember the following:

- A win is good for only one game. Don't get too cocky.

- You don't have to be perfect to win. Don't get down on yourself for an error or a strikeout.

- A game's not over until the final out is recorded. Never give up.

- Baseball is a game in which you can redeem yourself. Your final at-bat can erase that earlier error you made.

Baseball is a game through which players can learn about respect, hard work, teamwork, patience, persistence, and much more. It's also a game that teaches through defeat. Losses are never fun, but through a loss, players can learn the following:

- Sometimes you're better than the other team, and you still lose.

- Sometimes the other team is simply better than you.

- Sometimes you just have an off day, or you get unlucky.

- Sometimes you can work really hard and still lose.

Losing doesn't feel so hot. But remember the following:

- A loss is only for one game. Don't get too down.

- Pride comes before a fall. Don't chalk up a win before you take to the field.

- A game's not over until the final out is recorded. Never think you can coast home to victory.

THE ABSOLUTE MINIMUM

This chapter helped you consider all the issues involved in coaching during games. Among the key points were

- At the practice before the game, go over the game particulars—the field location, the time you want players to arrive, and so forth—and the game plan.

- Keep your tactics simple, especially at younger levels.

- Base your game plan and tactics on your team's strengths and abilities and on the opponent's weaknesses.

- Save the pregame speech. Just help your players focus on the fundamentals and game plan.

- Be aware of the signs of over-coaching and of under-coaching and steer toward a happy medium, being involved and encouraging but not directing your players' every move.

- Give your players guidance and technique tips, but don't overload them with information or corrections during games.

- Use score sheets to help you log information during games.

- Consider playing time issues and plan to give your players appropriate time on the field.

- At younger ages, move players around to various positions, but by age 9 or 10, have them focus on honing their skills at one or two positions.

- Display appropriate behavior at games. Remember that you are your players' role model.

- Lead your team in post-game handshakes with the opponents and hold a brief meeting afterward. Help your players take home positives from the game, regardless of the outcome.

- Help your players learn from both wins and losses.

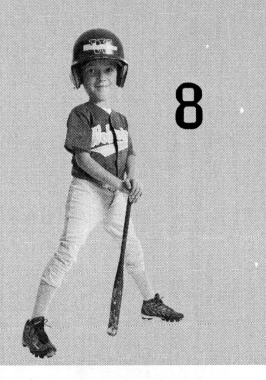

8

INGREDIENTS OF A SUCCESSFUL SEASON

The final game of the season is over and your players shake hands with the opponents. You hold a brief team meeting, and afterward, as most of the other team's players depart, many of your players hang around with their parents or friends, joking, playing catch, and having fun. Four of your players race around the bases to see who is fastest from home to home. You watch Chris, Dante, Kyle, and Ann tear around the bases, running off energy you wish you could bottle and store for yourself.

And you can't help but smile. "Hey, you goofballs!" you call out to the four speedsters. "You should have done a little more of that this season!"

To a casual observer, it would be hard to tell that your team had just lost its final game, 12-6, finishing with a 4-8 record. That casual observer might think, from the way your team is carrying on, that you just won the league championship.

You didn't, at least numbers-wise. You finished in the lower half of the pack. But baseball, with all its fascination for statistics, is so much more than numbers. And, for that matter, success at the youth level is so much more than winning percentages, league titles, and trophies.

There's nothing wrong, of course, with winning the league title or having a good winning percentage. In fact, that's what every team strives for. Those just aren't the only indicators of success, and you need to measure your accomplishments as a coach in other ways.

Why? There are many answers to that question, but two will suffice here. First, the hand you were dealt, in terms of player talent, doesn't always come up aces. Sometimes it comes up a mixture of low, unmatched cards. Second, the winning percentage or league trophy simply doesn't tell the complete story. Consider the following two cases.

A Tale of Two Coaches

The Tigers compiled a 10-2 regular season record and went on to win the Border League championship. Yet, after the title game, the players' celebration was strangely subdued, showing as much relief as joy. Coach McReady didn't take part in the celebration, but watched it with an air of satisfaction and pride. No player came over to congratulate Coach McReady, and he made no move to congratulate any player.

At a players-only pizza party that night, the conversation went like this:

"I'm glad that's over."

"Me too. I couldn't wait."

"I wonder what Coach McReady would have said if we lost?"

"Probably what he said after our two regular season losses, only ten times worse."

"I'm not playing next year."

"Me either."

"Why not?"

"Are you kidding? You want to go through that again?"

Coach McReady got the most out of his players' ability. He knew the game, he knew the skills and how to teach them, and he prepared his players to compete.

But he also trampled all over them emotionally and psychologically. Three players played the absolute minimum the league would allow. He yelled at players for making errors, the veins sticking out in his neck as he did, and he made players run laps and do pushups for every error they made. He cried out in disgust when they made outs in key situations, even if they hit a line drive. He screamed at his pitchers when they issued a walk or gave up a hit to what he called a "sissy" hitter. He berated the umpires; no one liked to umpire the Tigers' games.

No one caught him smiling all season long. His normal pose was off to the side, scowling, his arms folded across his thick chest, a critical look in his eye. He shouted harshly enough at four players to make them cry, and when they cried, he ridiculed them for being babies.

The Orioles, on the other hand, finished the regular season at 4-8 and got knocked out of the playoffs in the first round, losing 6-5 to the Tigers. (After that game, Coach McReady spent 10 minutes lambasting his players for almost getting beat by "a bunch of pansies" and told his players they might as well go home and play with their dolls if they couldn't play any better than that.)

The Orioles were disappointed that they were beaten, but they had a festive pizza party afterward, and the players presented Coach Giles with a "Coach of the Year" plaque.

Coach of the Year for a 4-8 team? Though it was not an official league award, it well could have been. Consider these items:

- All of Coach Giles's players were as happy and excited about baseball at the end of the season as they were at the beginning.
- All his players improved their skills throughout the season.
- They also gained in their understanding of the game's tactics and rules.
- The Orioles played hard every game, getting the most out of their abilities. They never gave up, and they didn't mope after losses.
- They pulled together as a team, rooting each other on, enjoying each other's successes, and encouraging each other after a failed attempt.
- The Orioles *did* win an official league title—the sporting behavior award as "Best Sports."
- Everyone played, everyone improved, and everyone had fun.

Of course, many championship teams are coached very well and are successful not only in their win-loss record, but also in the ways the Orioles were successful. That wasn't the case with the Tigers and Coach McReady, however.

Which coach would *you* rather be: Coach McReady or Coach Giles?

Evaluating Your Season

If winning isn't the only way to evaluate your success, what are the measures you should use? What are the keys to having a truly successful season? Throughout the rest of this chapter we focus on those keys. They shouldn't come as a surprise to you because they're a summation of everything you've learned in the first seven chapters.

These same keys provide the foundation for Appendix F, "Season Evaluation Form." After you read this chapter and complete your season, use Appendix F to evaluate your own season.

Did Your Players Have Fun?

As you'll recall from Chapter 1, "Your Coaching Approach," having fun is the main reason kids play baseball. That's an easy enough concept for most coaches to grasp before the season begins, but once the practices get underway, that concept can get lost amidst the more immediate and pressing goals and duties of a coach.

Can you win without having fun? Yes. But consider this: By the time kids reach age 13, their drop-out rate from sports is 75%. Some of that attrition is due to simply a lack of ability to compete at their age level anymore. Some of it is due to new interests that take up their time, such as music, art, or drama. But for the most part, players drop out of sports because

- They don't get enough playing time. Consistently when asked, kids respond they'd rather play for a losing team than sit on the bench for a winning team.
- They don't learn the skills they need to be competitive.
- They feel like failures (mainly because they haven't learned the skills). Their coaches don't reinforce their competence or help them see the positive aspects of their performance.
- They receive too much negative feedback from coaches.
- The sports environment is too negative; it's not enjoyable to go to practices or games.
- They stress out over winning because winning is overemphasized.
- Practices are poorly organized, tedious, and boring. Drills are repetitive, players are inactive, and the fun is drained out of the experience.

"Fun," then, doesn't mean telling jokes at practice, or goofing off, or trying to entertain your players. It means giving them playing time and building their skills so they'll feel competent when they have that playing time. It means reinforcing the skills they have and helping them focus on their positives, rather than dwelling on their negatives. It means giving them feedback but couching it in positive terms. It means making practices active, meaningful, and enjoyable, using a variety of games and drills that are game-like and that help them build their skills.

What are indications that your players are having fun? It's easy to see in the smiles on their faces, their body language, their focus, their effort, and their encouragement of each other.

Perhaps the greatest indication of all, though, is that they're happy at the end of the season, no matter what their record was and they can't wait for next baseball season to roll around.

Did Your Players Learn New Skills and Improve on Previously Learned Skills?

In considering player performances, all too often a season is judged on where the players ended, without regard to where they *began*. The true measure of success here is how much your players improved over the season. If they were good to begin with and ended up being good, without showing any real improvement, something went wrong. If they were poor to begin with and ended up being average, that's showing improvement.

Here are some of the mistakes coaches make in this area:

- They lack the teaching skills or technical know-how to help their players learn new skills or improve ones they've already learned.
- They are poor practice planners, meaning they squander their practice time or run ineffective drills.
- They push players to learn too fast or present advanced skills and tactics too early.
- They don't present advanced skills and tactics as the players develop; they keep them at an elementary level and don't help them hone skills.
- They focus on their better players and offer little help to their lesser-skilled players.

The best coaches can work with kids of varying abilities and help them all progress. They don't ignore their lesser-skilled players, and they adjust their teaching plan according to the skill levels of the kids, always gently pushing for improvement.

To foster such improvement, first you need to be able to plan and conduct effective practices. You also need a critical eye to assess talent and needs, the teaching skills to instruct and reinforce your players on the correct techniques, plenty of patience because players seem to sometimes take one step forward and two steps backward in learning, and the ability to encourage and support your players as they continue their growth.

Every season is a building season, an opportunity for players to become better, build on their talent and success, and come back for an even better year next year because they have deepened and broadened their abilities.

note

There's joy as a coach in watching good players perform up to their capabilities. There's even greater joy in helping lesser-talented players pick up skills and perform beyond where they or anyone else thought they were capable of performing.

Did You Help Your Players Understand the Game and Its Rules?

Lots of games are decided by players' physical skills—by their abilities to pitch, hit, field, throw, and run the bases.

And a lot of games are decided by players' abilities to apply the rules and execute the strategies: Alex forgets to tag up on a fly ball and a run is lost. Darnell doesn't realize a tag play is in order, thus allowing a runner to reach third base safely when he steps on the base instead of tagging the runner. This runner eventually scores the winning run. The list could go on and on.

It's tempting to focus solely on teaching skills because that's such an obvious need. But players, especially at the youth level, need to also grasp the bigger picture of how to perform those skills and how to use their abilities within the rules to benefit their team.

When you build the teaching of rules and strategies in to your drills and practice games, you are one step ahead of most coaches—and one step closer to building a competitive, savvy squad that knows how to play the game and does the little things that don't show up in a traditional box score. These little things can make the difference between winning and losing and between players enjoying the game and being confused or disappointed.

Did You Communicate Appropriately and Effectively?

Baseball fields across America are filled with coaches who know their stuff but don't know how to communicate it. Why? Because they think their ability to talk qualifies them as good communicators. (Of course, having read Chapter 3, "Communication Keys," you know this is far from the truth.)

Some of the signs of poor and ineffective communication include

■ Players don't learn skills because the coach can't communicate clearly.

■ Parents aren't kept informed and don't know how to pitch in and help.

- Players hang their heads or begin to miss practices because their coach yells at, degrades, or berates them.

- Players look bored or confused because their coach uses 100 words when 10 would suffice.

- Players don't listen to their coach because he doesn't speak with command or authority. This has nothing to do with volume or gruffness; it has everything to do with understanding, preparation, clarity, and delivery.

- Players aren't sure what to do in certain game situations because their coach hasn't told them.

- Players don't pay attention because their coach doesn't know how to get and hold their attention.

- Players appear wary and unsure because their coach said one thing but her body language said something different.

- Messages get lost, feelings get hurt, and sometimes tempers flare because the coach is too busy talking to listen to players or parents.

- Players, parents, and coaches become frustrated.

Your ability to communicate has significant impact on your overall coaching effectiveness. As you teach skills, do you clearly demonstrate them and use language your players can understand? As you correct errors and encourage players, what does your body language communicate, and is it in synch with your words? Do you *listen* to your players' comments and questions, and do you read and interpret their body language, as surely as they do yours?

> **note**
>
> Do you maintain control of your emotions as you communicate? Note that this doesn't mean you don't *show* emotion; it means you *control* it.

Did you communicate with parents before the season, letting them know your philosophy and coaching approach, your expectations of the players, and what the players and parents could expect of you? Are you maintaining a healthy flow of communication with parents as the season progresses?

Did You Provide for Your Players' Safety?

Providing for your players' safety doesn't mean no injuries happen on your watch. It means, ideally, that no *preventable* injuries happen and that whatever injuries *do* happen, you tend to them appropriately.

It's all in the planning and preparation. You plan for safety, you take the necessary precautions, and (when need be) you respond to the abrasion, bump, bruise, or twisted ankle when it occurs.

You are on your way to fulfilling your responsibilities here if you

- Are trained in CPR and first aid
- Have a well-stocked first aid kit on hand at practices and games, and know how to use it
- Make sure you know of any allergies or medical conditions of players, and know how to respond if the allergies or conditions flare up
- Warn your players and their parents of the inherent risks of baseball
- Check the practice and game fields for safety hazards and eliminate those hazards, if possible, before playing on the fields
- Enforce rules regarding equipment use and player behavior that enhance player safety
- Provide proper supervision throughout each practice
- Offer proper skill instruction
- Take a water break during practice
- Monitor your pitchers and allow them a maximum of 75 pitches per game

Did You Plan and Conduct Effective Practices?

If you played youth sports, you undoubtedly attended a practice or two in which your coach was winging it. His "preparation" time was spent driving to the practice field, and the drills he chose seemed to have no real purpose to them, other than to bore you to tears. You didn't learn any new skills or refine the ones you had; you simply spent time—and poorly, at that.

Have you spent time planning your season and your practices? Are you effective in running your practices? Signs of effectiveness include

- Kids pay attention to you because you have a purpose to what you're doing.
- There is no down time while you're trying to figure out what to do next.
- Players are active and engaged at multiple stations that you run simultaneously; they aren't standing around waiting for a turn.
- You use games and drills that are designed to teach a specific skill or tactic you want your players to work on that day.
- Your players are learning new skills and refining ones they have.
- Your players are having fun in practice.

There's one more sign you're planning and conducting well: *you're* having fun, too. When you're prepared and your practices have a purpose to them, it's enjoyable for everyone involved.

Did Your Players Give Maximum Effort in Practices and Games?

You might wonder why this question would be part of evaluating your success. After all, motivation comes from within; you can't make your kids try harder.

This is true. But you can create an environment that increases the likelihood your players will give full effort. Conversely, you can create an environment that stifles motivation.

Obviously, you want to do the former and not the latter. Before detailing the type of environment that motivates kids, let's consider the type of environment that leaves them high and dry.

Some of the ways a coach can demotivate players include

- Yelling at them for errors and for their general quality of play
- Comparing a child to a better player
- Having kids wait in line to take their turn
- Not teaching players the skills they need
- Appearing to not care about their performances or about them as individuals
- Playing favorites, and paying little attention to lesser-talented children
- Not listening to them

Some coaches mistakenly believe yelling is the best motivator. Their players do become motivated to behave in a way that makes their coach stop yelling, which, it might be argued, is the coach's point. But if you yell at a kid to keep his glove down, using an angry or irritated tone of voice, the child will often respond by becoming tense and anxious, which increases the likelihood that he'll make another mistake on the next ball hit to him.

Is it wrong to tell the player to keep his glove down? Not at all. It's wrong to yell it at him, showing your anger or irritation.

So, how do you create an environment in which your players are motivated to do their best? You do so by

- Teaching players the skills they need
- Giving kids specific technique goals to work toward
- Giving specific, positive feedback as players work on their skills
- Encouraging kids, especially when they get down, and praising correct technique and effort
- Helping kids take home the positives of the practice or game
- Praising hustle, desire, and teamwork shown in practice and games

- Running efficient, purposeful practices in which players are active and engaged the whole time
- Valuing each child for his or her own abilities and personality
- Caring about the kids as players and as children
- Listening to players

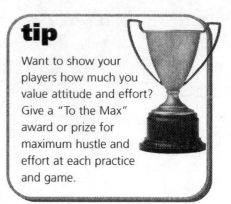

tip

Want to show your players how much you value attitude and effort? Give a "To the Max" award or prize for maximum hustle and effort at each practice and game.

When you create an environment in which your players are motivated to learn and perform, you'll reap the rewards in practices and games.

Did Your Players Leave the Games on the Field?

League games can be highly emotional events. The players are performing in front of parents, other family members, and their peers. They want to play well. They want to win. Many of them have dreams of becoming a major league player some day.

Then the ground ball scoots right between their legs. They strike out in a crucial situation. They overthrow a teammate. They walk in a run with the bases loaded. They drop an easy pop-up. They are called out at home when they're sure they were safe. They are playing against a team that likes to trash talk. They mount a comeback, only to fall short by one run in the final inning.

Individual failures and team losses are not easy to take, but all players have to learn how to deal with personal and team setbacks. Losing happens. In fact, it happens once a game. Kids have widely divergent reactions to losing. Often, at younger ages, you can't tell which team won by the responses and behaviors of both teams immediately following the game. Sometimes, though, defeats can have an impact on kids, no matter what age they are.

Realize that while they take many cues from you, they also are heavily influenced by their parents' views on winning and losing and by the cultural stigma attached to losing. Some kids take losing very personally; some feel it marks them somehow; some feel they let their teammates down; some respond by being poor sports; others don't know how to master the emotions that come with disappointment.

Part of your duty is to help them master those emotions, keep the game in perspective, and leave it (whether it was a win or a loss) on the field. They can't erase a loss, and they can't carry forward a win. They start out 0-0 in their next game.

Talk to your team before the first game about keeping the wins and losses in perspective, and then watch for players who are too high after a win or too low after a loss. Help your players keep a level head if they win a big game or play exceptionally well, and help them look forward to the next game if they lose or play poorly.

Did *You* Leave the Games on the Field?

Jerry was coaxed to coach the Pirates, his son Brandon's team, at the last minute. He went into the season with much trepidation because he had never coached before. But he found he liked it, and he had a good team and they played well—"in spite of the coaching they get," Jerry wryly told his friends.

They won their first three games, including an upset against the Cardinals, the league's best team from the previous year. The Cardinals had most of their players back.

The next game, though, the Pirates lost to the Reds, who weren't all that good. To his chagrin and surprise, Jerry didn't sleep very well that night. He couldn't believe he could lose sleep over a youth baseball game. But he did.

As the season went on, the Pirates and the Cardinals were running neck and neck for first place. They each accumulated three losses in the regular season, and Jerry took each loss harder than the previous loss.

"It's all right, Dad," Brandon told his dad on the way home after the Pirates' second loss.

After the third loss, Brandon said nothing on the way home because his dad was too upset. "There's no way we should have lost to the Cubs!" Jerry groused to no one in particular as he drove home. "That umpire had two different strike zones tonight. It was ridiculous."

That might have been true, but what was *more* ridiculous was Jerry's response to the loss. He not only didn't leave the game at the field, but also took it home with him, slept with it, and got up the next morning and dragged it to work with him.

It's easy to get wrapped up in the wins and losses, to care so much about the kids and want them to win so badly that you let the game's outcome affect you more than it should. Care about the outcome, yes. By all means care about the kids. But do what you want them to do: Leave it at the field and come prepared to the next practice to go forward, leaving behind any baggage from the last game.

Did You Conduct Yourself Appropriately?

As you know, you're a role model for your players. How good a model you are is up to you. A few signs of a good role model include

■ You communicate in positive ways with opposing coaches and players and with umpires.

■ You coach within the rules and have your players play within them.

■ You maintain control of your emotions in practices and games while providing the coaching and support your players need.

■ You keep the games in perspective and help your players do the same.

Remember this: Briefly losing your cool does not necessarily mean you failed as a role model. In fact, you can use such an instance to send a healthy message to your players. When you admit that you made a mistake and apologize for it, you set a positive example for the kids.

Did You Communicate Effectively with Parents and Involve Them in Positive Ways?

Some coaches put up with parents. Others look to placate them and hold them at bay. Still others do their best to ignore them, communicating with them as little as possible.

These coaches are missing the boat. At worst they are inviting trouble, and at the least they are overlooking a rich source of support and help.

Parents are your chief allies, and most parents want to help in some way, to make the sport experience as good as possible for their son or daughter. Yes, there are parents who present problems to coaches, but these are in the minority.

You read in Chapter 3 about ways to communicate with and involve parents. If you have healthy communication and involvement throughout the season, it probably looks something like this:

■ You have few or no misunderstandings with parents regarding your coaching philosophy.

■ You delegate responsibilities, sharing the workload with a lot of parents—and making your program stronger in doing so.

■ You aren't as stressed as you might be, had you not involved parents.

■ You appropriately address the few misunderstandings or concerns parents have.

When you have a good communication flow with parents and involve them in your program, everyone benefits.

Did You Coach Appropriately During Games?

Some coaches don't make the distinction between coaching in practices and coaching at games, and their players suffer for it. In Chapter 7, "Game Time!" you learned of the perils of over-coaching and under-coaching and the keys of effective coaching during games.

So, what does effective coaching during games look like? You get high marks for game-day coaching if most of these statements apply to your game days:

- You keep your strategy simple and base it on your players' strengths and abilities and on your opponent's weaknesses.
- You help your players get mentally prepared for the game by focusing them on the fundamentals they need to execute and on the game plan.
- You provide tactical direction and guidance throughout the game.
- You are encouraging and supportive.
- You give technique tips and reminders, and let the kids play, saving the error correction for the next practice.
- You tend to the kids' needs during the game—emotional and psychological as well as mental and physical.
- You help players keep the game in proper perspective.
- You use a positive coaching approach.
- You effectively rotate players in and out.
- Your players conduct themselves well during and after the game, including the post-game handshake.
- You hold a brief post-game meeting, giving the kids some positives to take home, regardless of the outcome of the game.

Coach games in a manner that helps kids develop their skills, learn the game, compete well, and enjoy the experience. When you do that, you're assured of a winning season, no matter what your record is.

Did You Win with Class and Lose with Dignity?

Many players learn how to hit, field, pitch, and run the bases. Plenty of players enjoy good seasons, and numerous teams enjoy superlative winning records.

Unfortunately, not all those players and teams learn how to handle their successes. Puffed up with their own accomplishments, they taunt or trash talk the other team during the game and celebrate the victory after the game in a way that rubs the loss in to the other team.

Your coaching duties don't end with teaching your team how to execute and how to compete and win. It extends to teaching them how to handle victories and defeats.

A prime example of winning with class and losing with dignity occurred during the 2004 National League Division Series between the St. Louis Cardinals and Los Angeles Dodgers. The Cardinals won the series 3 games to 1, and immediately after the last out of the final game, players from both teams met on the field, shaking hands and congratulating each other. It was a show of respect for both sides. The Dodgers held their heads up in losing and more than maintained their dignity, and the Cardinals, while celebrating their series win, handled themselves with class as they congratulated the Dodgers on their efforts and season.

Teach your players to win with the same class and to lose with the same dignity displayed at the end of that series. Winning and losing are part of life, and the lessons the players can learn through baseball can help them deal with wins and losses in other arenas throughout their lives.

Here's what winning with class looks like:

- You and your players shake hands with the other team, offering them congratulations.
- You thank the umpires for volunteering their time.
- Your team celebrates fully but in a way that shows respect for the other team.

And here's what losing with dignity looks like:

- Your players don't hang their heads, no matter how hard the loss was.
- You and your players congratulate the other team, looking them in the eye as you do.
- You thank the umpires for volunteering their time.
- You hold a brief team meeting and help the players regroup and take home positives from the game.

The ability to be gracious in victory and disappointed yet not defeated when you're on the short end of the score is all about character. You can help your players build character throughout the season, not only in games but in practices as well. Players can build character by having respect for themselves and others, by caring for others, by maintaining their integrity, and by following through on their responsibilities.

note

Kids can give their all on the field, but they can't control the outcome of the game. When you help your players build character, they will know how to win with class and lose with dignity.

Did You Make the Experience Positive, Meaningful, and Fun for Your Players?

This is what it all boils down to: Was the experience positive for your players? Was it fun? Did it leave them wanting to come back for more? Championships or winning records don't mean much if the players can't wait for the season to end and half of them don't return the next year for a repeat performance.

Was the season meaningful to your players? Did they learn the skills and tactics, the game, and the rules? Did they learn about themselves, how they respond to challenges, how to win, how to lose? Did they build character? For some telltale signs of a season that was positive, meaningful, and fun, see the following sidebar, "Signs of a Season Well Spent."

If your players show at the end of the season the same zest and enthusiasm that they showed at the beginning, you know you did well in this area. And you can look forward to welcoming them back next season.

SIGNS OF A SEASON WELL SPENT

Here are some signs of a memorable season. Hopefully, you will be able to identify with some of these signs when your season concludes:

- "Yeah, we were 5-7. We lost a couple of tough games, and we had a few games where we didn't play so well. But you know what? The kids improved over the season. They were really clicking and playing well at the end. And they had fun through it all." —*Coach Wilkens*

- "Cody was the worst hitter on our team throughout most of the season. He was afraid to hit. But he really blossomed at the end; he somehow gained the confidence to stand in there and hit, and he never gave up on himself. His technique improved dramatically from beginning to end. You should have seen the smile on his face when he started getting some hits! I had lots of kids who hit better, but I was happiest of all for Cody." —*Coach Yarborough*

- "I'd say, 'Molly, do you understand the tag-up rule?' and she'd say, 'Yes.' Then she'd run on a pop-up to the infield. I'd say, 'Molly, remember, you can't leave your base until a fly ball or pop-up has been caught.' And she'd say, 'Okay.' And she'd run immediately on a fly ball the next time, too. It took her half the season to get it. But she finally got it. I thought her teammates were going to lift her on their shoulders when she tagged up from third and scored on a fly ball!" —*Coach Mancini*

- "I just want to thank you for working so patiently with Andre. I know he gets distracted and he sometimes doesn't listen, or he forgets. Your patience made a big difference—and it showed in his play." —*Andre's mother*

- "I was really impressed with your practices; the team Jeremy was on last year wasn't run nearly so well. Jeremy learned so much more this year. Thanks, too, for letting me get involved. I really enjoyed helping you out." —*Jeremy's father*

- "Thanks for being a good role model for DeShawn. He's so competitive and he *hates* to lose. It's easy for his temper to get the best of him. The way you kept your cool during games really showed him something. Every time he wanted to blame an umpire or complain about the other team, you focused his attention on his own performance. I think he really grew up this season. Thank you!" —*DeShawn's mother*

- "Hey, Coach, is there a fall league?" —*Your players*

The Absolute Minimum

This chapter focused on the ingredients of a successful season. That success can be evidenced in a good win-loss record, but that just scratches the surface. Digging a little deeper, true success in a baseball season is evidenced by these signs:

- Your players learned the skills, tactics, and rules they needed to know to compete to the best of their abilities.

- Your players were mentally, emotionally, and physically ready to play each game.

- Your players improved their skills and understanding of the game over the season.

- Your players had fun at practices and games.

- Your players displayed good sporting behavior throughout the season.

- You communicated appropriately with everyone involved—players, parents, umpires, and league administrators—and involved parents in your program.

- You planned and conducted practices effectively, keeping players actively engaged and presenting skills in a logical order.

- You taught skills and tactics effectively, showing and demonstrating how they should be performed and putting kids in game-like situations to practice the tactics and skills.

- Your players gave maximum effort in practices and games.

- You provided the coaching the kids needed during the games.

- You and your players gave each game your best and, win or lose, you all were able to leave the game on the field and keep the outcome in perspective.

- You taught your players to win with class and lose with dignity and guided them in doing so, leading by example.

PART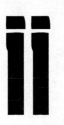

Skills and Tactics

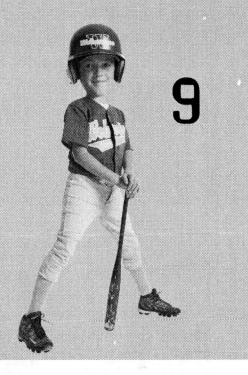

9

OFFENSIVE SKILLS AND TACTICS

In Chapter 5, "Practice Plans," you learned about planning your season and your individual practices, and in Chapter 6, "Player Development," you learned the method of teaching skills. Now, in the next two chapters, you'll be presented with the mechanics for all the skills and tactics you'll need to teach. Then, in Chapter 11, "Games and Drills," you'll find games and drills you can use to teach the skills and tactics.

In this chapter, the focus is on offensive skills and tactics—hitting, bunting, and baserunning. Use this chapter to learn about the proper execution of offensive skills and tactics and to refresh your memory before you teach the skills and tactics to your players.

Hitting

Hitting a thrown ball is one of the most difficult skills to learn, and to teach, in sports. Just look at it this way: At the major league level, hitters are considered quite accomplished if they manage to *fail*—that is, to not get a hit—7 out of 10 times!

As you watch major league hitters, you'll notice a variety of hitting styles. Some have wide stances, some hold the bat high above their head, some crouch, some stand close to the plate, and some stand far away. But they all approach the fundamentals in the same way.

Likewise, your hitters might have different styles at the plate. Your job isn't to make everyone look identical at the plate, but to help each player learn and execute the fundamental techniques all good hitters need to master.

The first thing your hitters have to do is select a bat that is a good weight and length for them. In the following sections you'll learn about bat selection, and then you'll explore the five main components of hitting: grip, stance, picking up the pitch, stride, and swing.

Bat Selection

Encourage your players to experiment with several different bats in practice before choosing the one that best suits them. Some bats have thicker handles than others, and bat lengths and weights differ. Players should choose a bat that feels good to them, that they can grip well, and that they can generate good bat speed with.

Choking up on a bat can help a player offset using a heavier or longer bat. A player chokes up by moving his hands up from the bottom end of the bat, so that a few inches show below his grip.

If your players appear to have trouble swinging the bat, steer them toward a lighter bat.

Grip

Teach players to use a relaxed grip. They should hold the bat firmly in their fingers, with their middle knuckles lined up (see Figure 9.1). Make sure they don't grip the bat only with their palms. The grip naturally tightens some as hitters begin their swing.

FIGURE 9.1
A proper grip, with the knuckles lined up.

Stance

You'll see greater variety in stance than in any other aspect of hitting. Although there is no single correct stance, you can guide players in finding the stance that works best for them. Following are some aspects to consider.

Comfort

Hitters won't be successful if they aren't comfortable in the batter's box. Comfort entails a lot of things, including the type of stance they use, how close to the plate they are, how deep in the box they stand, and how they position themselves. Don't try to force a player to use a stance that works for another hitter; focus on working on the proper mechanics in the stance that each hitter is most comfortable in.

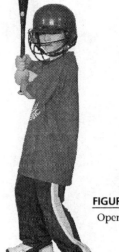

FIGURE 9.2
Open stance.

Location in Batter's Box

The only rule regarding location is that hitters must be completely in the batter's box (the lines are part of the box). Beyond that, batters can stand as close to or as far from the plate as they want and as deep in the box (nearer the catcher) or up (nearer the pitcher) as they desire.

Location is largely a matter of preference and comfort. Make sure players don't stand so close that they get jammed with inside pitches or so far away that they can't cover the outer part of the plate. For faster pitchers, hitters might want to stand a little deeper in the box to give themselves a little more time to swing.

Type of Stance

There are three basic types of stances: open, closed, and squared.

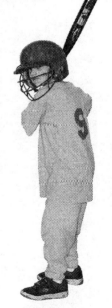

FIGURE 9.3
Closed stance.

In an *open* stance, a right-handed batter's lead foot (left foot) is farther away from the plate than the back foot is (see Figure 9.2). Thus, the hitter's body is opened up more to the pitcher.

In a *closed* stance, a right-handed batter's lead foot is closer to the plate than the back foot is (see Figure 9.3). Thus, the hitter's body is closed, or turned away from, the pitcher.

In a *squared* stance, both feet are the same distance from home plate (see Figure 9.4).

If players have no preference, a squared stance is a good stance to use, but if players are more comfortable in an open or a closed stance, that's fine, too, so long as the stance isn't extreme.

Body Position and Bat Angle

There are many things to watch for as players position themselves in the box:

- Both feet should be parallel with the back line of the batter's box. The feet should be about shoulder-width apart or a little wider, and the weight should be on the balls of the feet.

- The knees should be slightly bent, with a little more of the body weight supported on the back leg.

- The hands should be near the top of the strike zone (about chest height), slightly behind the back shoulder.

- The upper body should be slightly bent at the waist, with the elbows away from the body and pointed toward the ground.

- The bat should be held at a 45° angle to the ground.

See Figure 9.5 for a player in good position, ready to hit.

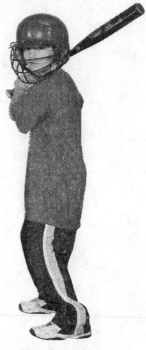

FIGURE 9.4

Squared stance.

Picking Up the Pitch

Teach your players to pick up the pitch as soon as it leaves the pitcher's hand. To do this, tell them to focus on the glove as the pitcher prepares to pitch because that's where the ball is. As the pitching arm comes toward the plate, and before the pitcher releases the ball, the hitter focuses on the hand and the ball and tracks its flight toward home.

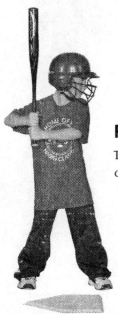

FIGURE 9.5

Batter in position, ready to hit.

Stride

Timing is critical to a hitter's success. As the pitcher prepares to release the ball, the hitter prepares to swing by transferring his weight more fully to the back leg. The hitter moves his hands back 3"–4" and closes his front shoulder, hip, and knee, moving them inward toward the back of the plate (see Figure 9.6). This inward movement is called *coiling*, and it prepares the batter to stride and swing.

Stride is another factor that can vary from player to player. Some players make a small stride toward the pitcher—that is, they pick up their front foot and move it laterally a few inches at a 45° angle toward home plate in preparing to swing (see Figure 9.7). Others pick up the front foot and drop it back down in the same spot before swinging. Neither is wrong (though a common mistake is to over stride; see "Common Errors in Hitting," later in this chapter). Either way, the hitter should plant the front foot before making contact with the ball. Instruct players to land on their big toe or on the inside of their front foot, stepping softly down as they prepare to swing.

As hitters stride, they should keep their weight back on their back leg. The front foot stays closed during the stride, not opening up toward the pitcher. If it opens up, it will cause the hitter's hips to open up too soon, and power will be lost in the swing.

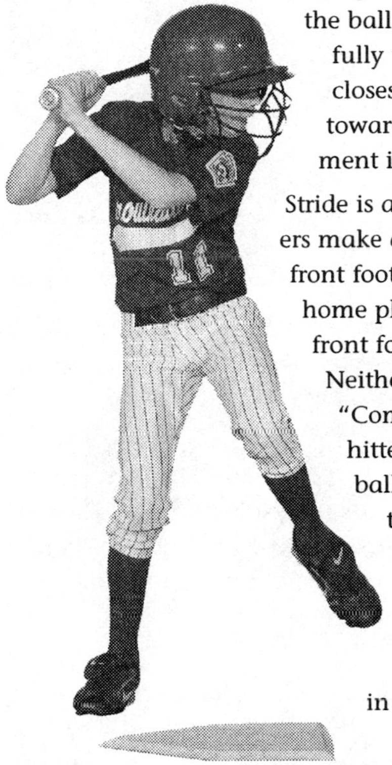

FIGURE 9.6

Batter coils in preparation to hit.

FIGURE 9.7

The front foot moves a few inches at a 45° angle toward home plate.

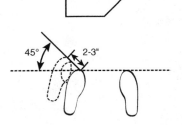

Swing

Many youngsters think their arms are the driving force behind their swing, but they're wrong. Their legs and hips drive the swing.

As a hitter plants his front foot, ending his stride, he transfers about 60% of his weight to his front leg. The front foot doesn't pivot, and the front leg remains stiff (see Figure 9.8).

The back foot pivots toward the pitcher as the front foot is planted, and the back hip drives the hips open toward the pitcher (see Figure 9.9). How far they open depends on the pitch location; for an outside pitch, they won't open as much. On inside pitches, hitters need to open their hips more to allow their hands to drive through the hitting zone.

The hands should be at the top of the strike zone when hitters begin their swing. If the hands are lower, hitters are likely to pop the ball up on a high strike.

Teach hitters to bring their hands through close to their body as they begin their swing. The lead elbow points toward the ground. The hands remain close on inside pitches; on outside pitches, the hands extend some. The barrel of the bat is above the hands during the swing and moves through the hitting zone parallel to the ground, or slightly downward.

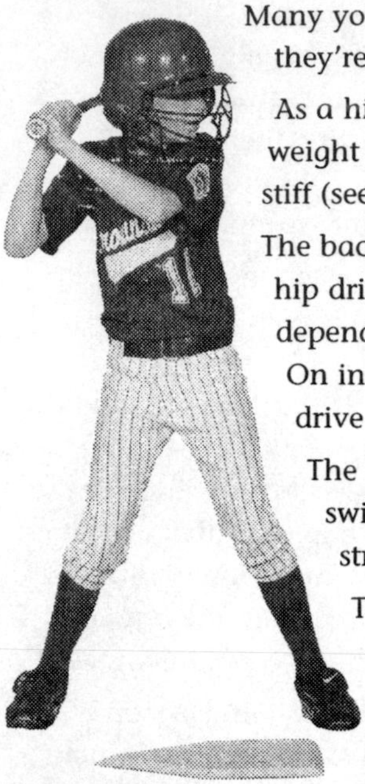

As hitters make contact, their bottom hand is palm down, their upper hand palm up. They should try to hit down and drive through the ball with a quick bat (see Figure 9.10). As the hands continue forward, the top hand comes off the bat as the bottom hand completes the follow-through (see Figure 9.11).

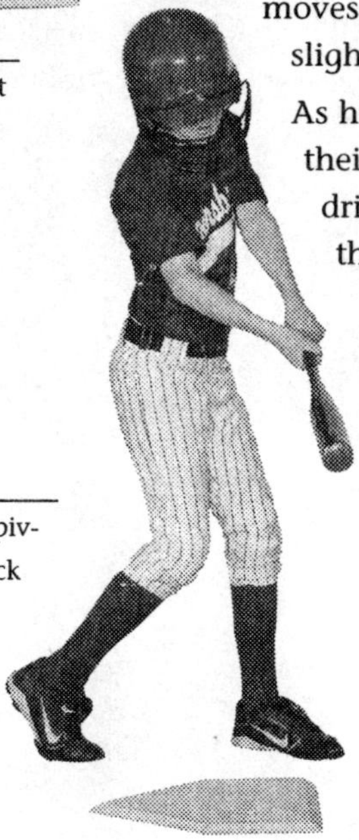

FIGURE 9.8
The front foot doesn't pivot, and the front leg remains stiff.

FIGURE 9.9
The back foot pivots and the back hip drives the hips open.

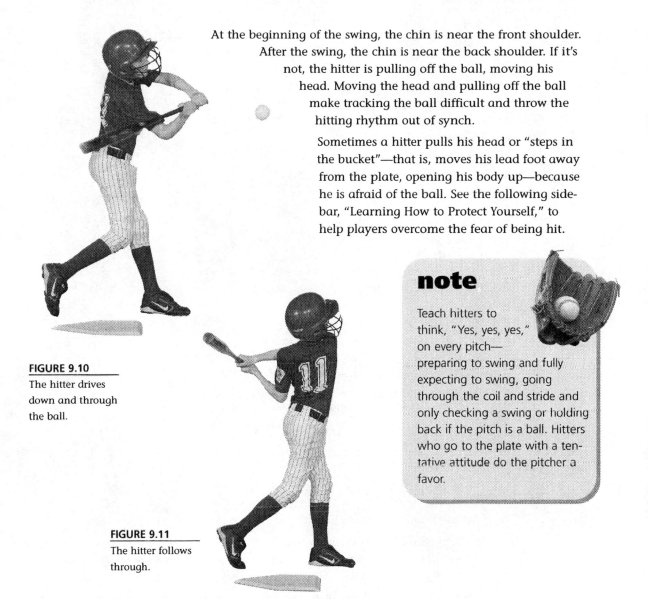

At the beginning of the swing, the chin is near the front shoulder. After the swing, the chin is near the back shoulder. If it's not, the hitter is pulling off the ball, moving his head. Moving the head and pulling off the ball make tracking the ball difficult and throw the hitting rhythm out of synch.

Sometimes a hitter pulls his head or "steps in the bucket"—that is, moves his lead foot away from the plate, opening his body up—because he is afraid of the ball. See the following side-bar, "Learning How to Protect Yourself," to help players overcome the fear of being hit.

FIGURE 9.10
The hitter drives down and through the ball.

note

Teach hitters to think, "Yes, yes, yes," on every pitch—preparing to swing and fully expecting to swing, going through the coil and stride and only checking a swing or holding back if the pitch is a ball. Hitters who go to the plate with a tentative attitude do the pitcher a favor.

FIGURE 9.11
The hitter follows through.

LEARNING HOW TO PROTECT YOURSELF

There's nothing worse as a hitter than going to the plate and being afraid of the ball. It's natural to have some fear of the ball, and that fear is accentuated by the wildness of many young pitchers. Often, if a young hitter is hit once or twice early in a season, he might shy away from the plate, pull his head or lead foot out, and develop other bad habits that essentially take the bat out of his hands.

Watch for hitters who might have developed this fear and help them overcome it. Teach them how to protect their bodies when a pitch is coming at them. Many young hitters simply back up, still standing tall; this doesn't protect the body at all. Instead, they should turn their bodies away from the ball, bending at the waist, so the ball has less of a target to hit. A ball above the waist will glance off the body rather than striking it full force (see Figure 9.12).

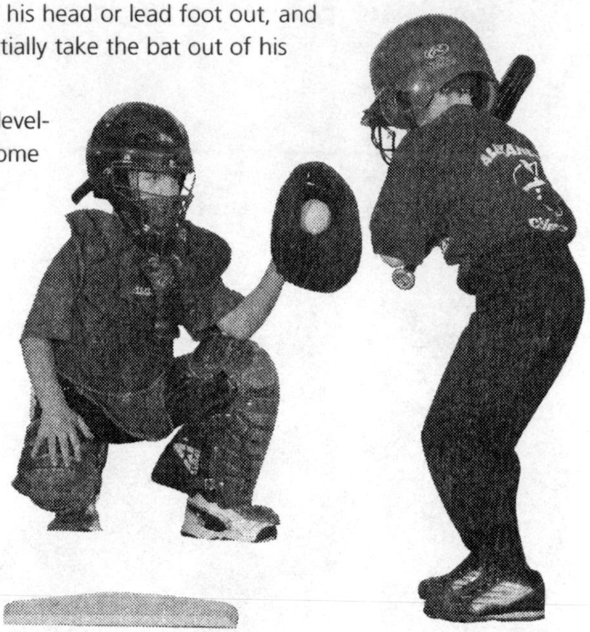

Incorporate a drill with hitters in which they practice getting out of the way of errant pitches and protecting themselves. Use tennis balls or some other type of soft ball and coach players on how to protect themselves, giving them plenty of practice in doing so. Then they'll be able to stride to the plate with more confidence, which is half the battle in hitting.

FIGURE 9.12
The hitter turns away from the pitch and bends down.

Common Errors in Hitting

Look for these common errors in hitting and help your players correct them:

- **The stance is too wide or too narrow**—With too wide a stance, the hitter loses power. With too narrow a stance, the hitter tends to over-stride. Instruct the hitter to stand with his feet about shoulder-width apart or slightly wider.

- **The hitter wraps the bat around her shoulders**—This results in a long or looping swing, and it is hard for the hitter to get the bat around in time to meet the pitch. Have the hitter hold the bat at a 45° angle off her back shoulder, angled slightly back, not wrapped around the shoulder.

- **The head is not turned far enough toward the pitcher**—This prevents the batter from getting a good view of the pitch. The hitter should be able to see the pitch with both eyes. Instruct him to turn his head more fully to the pitcher until he can easily see the pitcher with both eyes.

■ **The hitter's stride is too long**—This results in a late swing because the stride triggers the swing. Work with the hitter on striding no more than 2" or 3" and on beginning the stride sooner, if necessary.

■ **The hitter swings before she completes her stride**—The hitter will have no power even if she connects if her front foot is not planted. The stride should trigger the swing, not be performed simultaneously with it. Have the hitter take many practice swings on the side, swinging at an imaginary pitch, as you repeat, "Stride-swing" with each practice cut.

■ **The hitter has a hitch in his swing**—A *hitch* means the batter drops his hands and then picks them up again as he begins his swing. This delays the swing and causes the batter to be late. Instruct the hitter to move his hands slightly up and then back rather than dropping them. By moving up and back a bit, he moves the bat into the position where he has been putting it with the hitch, thus eliminating the hitch move to get the bat into that position.

■ **The hitter has an uppercut in his swing**—An uppercut results in pop-ups and fly balls. The best cut is level or even slightly down on the ball. Have the hitter focus on hitting the top half of the ball and on holding his hands at upper-chest level to begin his swing.

■ **The hitter opens her hips too soon**—This makes reaching the outer half of the plate difficult and drains power from the hitter. The batter's hips should open up in synch with her bat.

■ **The hitter steps in the bucket (see Figure 9.13)**—This often is a result of being afraid of the ball. The batter can't reach the outer half of the plate, diminishes his power, and pops up a lot of what he does reach. Work with the hitter on knowing how to get out of the way of errant pitches (refer to the sidebar "Learning How to Protect Yourself"), and focus him on making either a short stride at a 45° angle *toward* home plate or no stride at all. In the latter case, he should just focus on picking up his front foot and planting it in the same place it was.

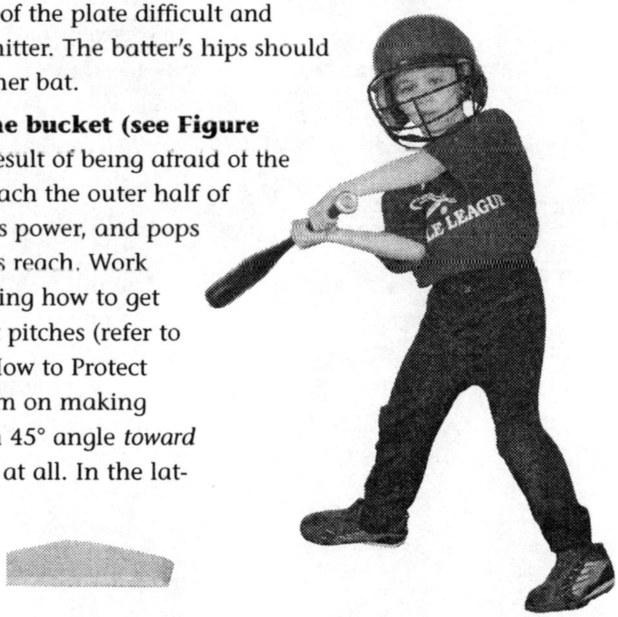

FIGURE 9.13

ERROR: The hitter steps in the bucket, away from the plate.

Bunting

There are many types of bunts: a straight sacrifice, to move the runner or runners along; a safety squeeze or suicide squeeze, to score a runner from third base; and a drag bunt or push bunt, to try to surprise the opponent and reach base. In this section you'll learn the technique for each type of bunt, as well as some common errors to look for and ways to correct the errors as your players attempt to master the skill of bunting.

> **tip**
>
> Coaches call for a sacrifice bunt in a variety of situations. When your team is facing a tough or overpowering pitcher and you're trying to manufacture runs and when you have a weaker hitter at the plate and need to move a runner along are two such situations. But don't automatically have your weaker hitters bunt; otherwise, they'll never get better as hitters.

Sacrifice Bunt

There are two methods that you can teach: squaring around or pivoting. If you're unsure of which method to use, practice both techniques for awhile and see which one, if either, your players are more proficient at. You can teach your players both methods or either method exclusively.

Squaring Around

When a batter squares around to bunt, he isn't trying to deceive the defense, though he still doesn't want to tip his hand too early. Thus, he squares around—pivots on the front foot and moves the back foot up with a quick jab step, placing it nearly parallel with the front foot—as the pitcher begins his windup (see Figure 9.14). The weight is on the balls of the hitter's feet.

The batter bends his knees and brings his top hand toward the trademark, gripping the bat between the index finger and thumb. He either keeps his bottom hand near the knob of the bat or slides it about 6" up (see Figure 9.15). With this grip, the ball won't be able to hit the bunter's top hand.

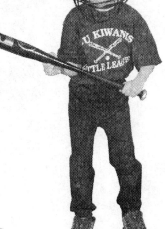

FIGURE 9.14

The hitter squares around to bunt, with feet nearly parallel and facing the pitcher.

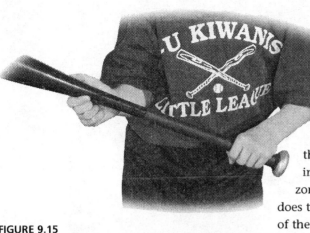

As shown in Figure 9.16, the batter holds the bat out in front of him, with the barrel angled up at the top of the strike zone (the crouch brings the batter lower than normal). The bunter's arms are in front of his body, slightly bent. The bat position and angle shown in Figure 9.15 give the bunter the best view of the pitch coming in. Holding the bat at the top of the strike zone, with the barrel higher than the knob, does two things: It helps the bunter know the top of the strike zone and helps him to bunt down on the ball, rather than pop it up.

FIGURE 9.15

Proper positioning of the hands. Note that the bottom hand can be kept near the knob or moved up the bat about 6".

FIGURE 9.16

The barrel is angled up and held at the top of the strike zone.

After getting into position, the batter adjusts to the pitch as it's coming in, bending at the knees and waist and lowering the bat to reach a low strike. The barrel should still be slightly above the handle as contact is made, and no matter where the pitch is, if the batter offers at it, he should attempt to contact the top half of the ball with his bat, so the ball will drop to the ground.

The angle of the bat from knob to barrel determines the direction the bunt will go. A right-handed hitter can drop a bunt down toward the third base side by holding the knob close to the body. A right-hander can bunt on the first base side by holding the knob farther away from the body.

> **tip**
>
> Teach batters to only bunt strikes! They should not offer at a pitch that is higher than the barrel of their bat. When they hold their bat at the top of the strike zone, anything above the barrel is a ball.

Contacting the ball is the final skill in bunting. After your players have developed the proper grip, stance, and bat angle, teach them to try to "catch" the ball with the bat, letting the ball come to the bat rather than pushing at the ball. Letting the ball come to the bat deadens the ball; pushing at it sends it sharply to the infield, where a play can be made more quickly.

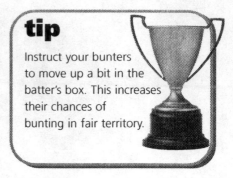

tip

Instruct your bunters to move up a bit in the batter's box. This increases their chances of bunting in fair territory.

The batter gets into his bunting position as the pitcher begins his motion to the plate, or shortly before.

Pivoting

Pivoting is another method of bunting. With this method, the batter pivots with the front foot and takes a short jab step toward the plate with the back foot. The rest of the technique—the grip, bat position and angle, and contact with the ball—is the same as it is in squaring away.

Safety Squeeze Bunt

A *safety squeeze* is used as a sacrifice bunt to score a runner from third base. The batter executes this bunt the same as she does any other sacrifice bunt, either squaring away or pivoting and using the techniques described in "Sacrifice Bunt."

The strategy behind a safety squeeze is simple: Score the runner. While it's ideal that the batter beats out the bunt, a coach is happy if the bunt gets down and the runner scores. The runner on third doesn't break for home on the pitch but gets a lead off of third and breaks for home the moment he sees that the bunt is down.

Because it isn't executed with the batter getting a hit in mind, a safety squeeze is used only when there are no outs or one out. It's called a *safety squeeze* because it's not very risky; the runner doesn't break unless he sees the bunt is down. If the batter misses the bunt, no harm is done (unless it's strike three). However, a safety squeeze puts pressure on the batter to lay down a *good* bunt because a bunt directly at the pitcher or the charging first or third baseman can often result in the runner being thrown out at the plate.

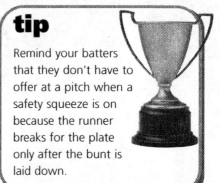

tip

Remind your batters that they don't have to offer at a pitch when a safety squeeze is on because the runner breaks for the plate only after the bunt is laid down.

As with the straight sacrifice bunt, the batter gets into her bunting position as the pitcher begins his motion to the plate, or shortly before.

Suicide Squeeze Bunt

The *suicide squeeze* is similar to the safety squeeze. In fact, there's no change for the batter. He gets into position at the same time, he executes the bunt in the same way, and his goal is the same—to get the bunt down and score the runner. The difference with the suicide squeeze is in how the runner on third approaches the play. She breaks for the plate as soon as the pitcher has committed to the plate; for her there's no turning back. If the batter misses the pitch and the catcher catches it, the runner is either easily out at the plate or caught in a rundown between third and home.

This bunt, then, puts pressure on the batter to get the ball down or even to foul off a poor pitch to protect the runner. The batter doesn't have to worry so much about where he bunts the ball; any fair bunt laid on the ground should easily score the runner.

note

Remind your batters when they're in a suicide squeeze situation that they *must* bunt the ball. They should attempt to make contact whether the pitch is a strike or ball.

Drag Bunt

The *drag bunt*, unlike the sacrifice bunt, is used in hopes of getting on base. Also unlike the sacrifice, a drag bunt is not shown until the last instant to catch the defense unaware and thus increase the chances of reaching base safely.

A batter approaches a drag bunt situation as if she were hitting away (taking a full swing). She should take her practice cuts and then stand in the box as she normally does when hitting away, although she might want to inch forward slightly in the box without tipping her hand. The method of bunting depends on whether the batter is left-handed or right-handed.

caution

Drag bunts and push bunts are harder to execute than sacrifice bunts. Your players should master the art of sacrifice bunting before moving on to drag and push bunting. Players under the age of 10 should focus only on basic bunting skills, not on drag or push bunting.

Left-handed Hitter

A left-hander drags the ball down the first base side. As the pitch comes in, the batter steps with his right foot toward the pitcher, brings the bat into position, and angles the contact so the ball goes on the first base side. This is accomplished by bringing the barrel of the bat forward and pointing it toward third base (see Figure 9.17). The best drag bunts are close to the line.

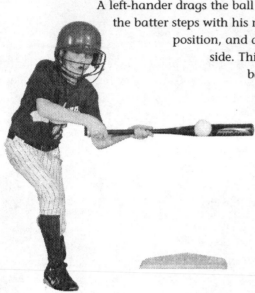

Unlike the sacrifice, the batter doesn't come to a set position before bunting; instead, he times the contact so that he can make a crossover step with his left foot and be in motion as the ball hits the bat.

Again, batters should offer only at pitches that are good to bunt. For a left-hander, these are pitches from the middle of the plate to the inner portion. As his body motion is going toward first, pitches on the outer part of the plate are hard to reach.

FIGURE 9.17
A left-handed hitter drags a bunt.

Right-handed Hitter

A right-hander drags a bunt by pulling his right foot back, bringing his bat into position, and angling the contact so the ball goes down the third base side. This is done by bringing the barrel forward and pointing it toward first base (see Figure 9.18). Ideally the bunt is close to the line.

A good pitch for the right-handed hitter to try to drag is anything from the middle part of the plate to the outside portion. As in any

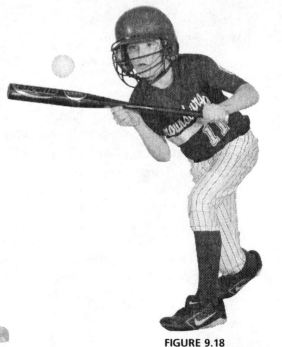

FIGURE 9.18
A right-handed hitter drags a bunt.

bunting attempt, the batter shouldn't offer at a pitch that is higher than his bat when it's in bunting position.

Push Bunt

Like the drag bunt, the *push bunt* is executed in an attempt to get a hit. Unlike the drag bunt, in which the batter is in motion while he's bunting, the push bunter does not begin running until he has bunted the ball. Most batters want to run right away when they're bunting for a base hit, so instruct your players to focus on getting the ball down before running on push bunts.

It's called a *push bunt* because, unlike in the sacrifice bunt, the batter actually pushes his bat toward the ball on contact. A right-handed hitter pivots and tries to push the ball past the pitcher and toward the second baseman. Usually, if the ball gets past the pitcher, the batter can beat out the bunt, unless it's hit too hard. The second baseman has to charge the ball hard; field it cleanly; and make a quick, accurate throw across his body to get the batter.

A left-handed hitter pivots and angles his bat so that he pushes the ball down the third base line.

Common Errors in Bunting

Here are some common errors in bunting and ways to correct them:

- **The batter drops only the barrel of the bat to reach a low strike, resulting in popping the ball up**—Instruct the batter to bend at the waist and knees, and if she has to lower the bat, she should lower both ends, not just the barrel.

- **The batter, in gripping the bat, exposes her top hand to the ball**—Show the hitter how to grip the bat so that the fingers and thumb are not exposed to the pitch.

- **The batter offers at pitches that are too high and pops them up**—Have the batter crouch and hold the bat at eye level, which should be the top of the strike zone. Have her practice bunting high strikes and not offering at pitches that come in higher than the bat.

- **The batter squares around too early, tipping her hand**—The hitter should wait till the last moment on a drag or push bunt before getting into bunting position. On sacrifices, she should move into position after the pitcher begins his motion toward home (or is near the end of his windup, if the pitcher is using a full windup).

- **The batter pivots too far with the back foot and steps on home plate or out of the batter's box in squaring around**—Remind your hitter to be aware of where the plate and box are and to keep her pivot short enough that it doesn't go beyond the box. Practice getting the pivoting part down before practicing the entire bunt technique.

- **The batter pushes at the ball with the bat on a sacrifice bunt, thus allowing the defense to field the ball more quickly**—Instruct the bunter to let the ball come to the bat and to try to deaden the ball. Tell the bunter to think of it as if she's catching the pitch with her bat.

- **The batter moves out the box before laying down the bunt**—This happens most often on drag bunts. The batter will be called out if she makes contact with the ball while either foot has touched the ground beyond the box. Remind the batter to focus on the contact first.

- **The batter bunts at a pitch that isn't a strike or that is difficult to bunt successfully**—This is appropriate only on a suicide squeeze to protect the runner racing to the plate. Otherwise, the batter should be just as selective in offering at only good pitches to bunt as she is at swinging at good pitches to hit. Remind her what constitutes a good pitch to bunt and practice by making both good and almost-good pitches to her; she needs to lay off the latter.

- **The batter crosses over too early with the back foot in dragging a bunt down the first base side**—This is a timing play and the early crossover is done in the batter's haste to make it to first. Again, help the batter focus on getting the ball down first, even as she is getting into position to run. It's more important to get this bunt down than to get a super jump.

Baserunning

Baserunning is a complex set of skills often overlooked in practice. Especially at younger levels, player confusion is often most evident on the base paths, with baserunners either running unnecessarily into outs or not taking advantage of opportunities to advance.

On the other hand, teams that are well-coached in baserunning can manufacture runs and help their cause with heads-up running. Relatively weak hitters can enhance their value to the team by being skillful baserunners.

Take the time, then, to teach your players the rules, skills, and tactics of baserunning. Make sure, of course, that you are clear on your league's baserunning rules because these are often modified to make the game most appropriate for younger and lesser-skilled players.

In this section you'll find an array of skills your players will need to learn, including

- Running from home to first
- Taking leadoffs
- Sliding
- Running from first to second
- Taking an extra base
- Running from third to home
- Stealing
- Hit-and-run
- Tagging up

At the end of the section you'll find common errors in baserunning and how to correct them.

Running from Home to First

For some hitters, the transition from batter to runner is not a smooth one. Unfortunately, a split second lost in starting from home to first can be the difference between being safe or out.

Here are the main points to get across to your players about running from home to first:

- Take a full swing, including your follow-through; then drop the bat and run. Don't cut your follow-through short in an attempt to quickly get out of the box.

- Drive out of box, using a quick jab step to start, driving low like a sprinter coming out of the starting blocks.

- Sprint all the way down the line. Don't look at the ball to see whether an infielder picked it up cleanly; just sprint. If the ball is in the air to the outfield, you can sneak a peek at it because you know that won't

note

Many younger runners don't run through the bag because they don't understand they are allowed to run past first base. Teach them that batter/runners can run past the bag without risking being tagged out unless they turn toward second base. Tell them to always turn to their right (toward foul territory) before they return to first base.

cause you to be thrown out at first, but you should still run at top speed, ready to take the extra base if possible.

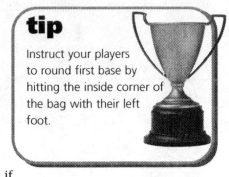

- Run *through* the bag, not *to* it. Don't slide into the base, and don't lunge for it or jump on it. Running through the base is the quickest way to reach it.

- If you hit a ground ball to the infield, be ready to advance to second on the first base coach's directions. This could happen if an infielder overthrows the first baseman.

- On a hit to the outfield, round first base by veering out slightly as you near the bag, then making a sharp cut at the bag. Run about a quarter to a third of the way to second, depending on how deep the ball is, and be ready to advance if the outfielder doesn't field the ball cleanly or makes a poor throw to the infield.

- Listen to the first base coach and make a full effort on every run. An infielder could bobble your grounder or make a weak throw. Even if this doesn't happen, you owe it to your team to give full effort on every play.

Taking Leadoffs

If your league allows leadoffs, you need to coach your players in how to take them. Too big a lead can cause a runner to be picked off the base. Too short a lead can cause a runner to be out on a bang-bang play in which he otherwise might have been safe.

Instruct your runners to take the longest lead they can take without being thrown out on a pickoff attempt. Practice pickoffs so your runners get a feel for what's safe for them and what's not. Of course, this differs depending on the skill of the pitcher in getting the ball quickly to first base.

As a runner takes his leadoff, he should always watch the pitcher, ready to get back to the base if the pitcher throws over. As the runner takes his lead, his shoulders are squared to the infield and his feet are a little wider than shoulder-width apart (see Figure 9.19). The knees are slightly bent, arms hanging down and loose. The runner shouldn't lean toward second base; in doing so, it is harder to return to first on a pickoff attempt.

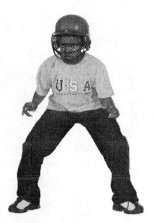

FIGURE 9.19

Taking a lead off of first base.

After the pitcher begins his delivery, the runner should take a secondary lead—two shuffle steps toward second base. This gives him momentum toward the base.

Sliding

Not knowing how to slide correctly causes numerous injuries in youth baseball. Players slide too late and jam their ankles or knees when they contact the bag; they slide on the side of their legs, and come home with scrapes and bruises; or they slide headfirst and jam their fingers on the base.

When players know how to slide correctly, they not only minimize the chance of being injured on the play, but also maximize their chance of being safe.

There are two main factors to teach in sliding: when to slide and how to slide.

When is it appropriate to slide? A player should slide if a play is going to be close at a base. The only exception is for the batter/runner running to first base. This is an exception because the batter/runner is allowed to run past the bag.

Base coaches should be watching the play and directing the runner on whether to slide, giving the direction well in advance of the need to slide.

note

Many leagues ban headfirst sliding. Even if yours doesn't, don't teach it, except in diving back to first base on a pickoff attempt. Why? Studies show that more injuries occur with headfirst sliding, and, despite the popular perception that headfirst sliding is faster than feet-first sliding, it is actually slightly slower at all levels of play from youth leagues through colleges.

Here's how you should instruct your players in performing a bent-leg slide (see Figure 9.20):

1. Start the slide about 6–8 feet from the bag.

2. Bend your knees and drop your hips toward the ground as you approach the bag. Place one leg under you so that your legs form a 4 (or a backward 4) as you slide. (Players should bend under them whichever leg feels more natural to bend.)

3. As you bend one leg under you, extend the other leg toward the base.

4. Slide on your buttocks, *not* the sides of your legs!

5. Keep your hands in the air. They shouldn't touch ground at all during the slide.

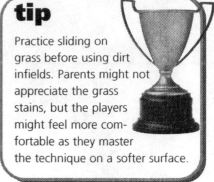

tip

Practice sliding on grass before using dirt infields. Parents might not appreciate the grass stains, but the players might feel more comfortable as they master the technique on a softer surface.

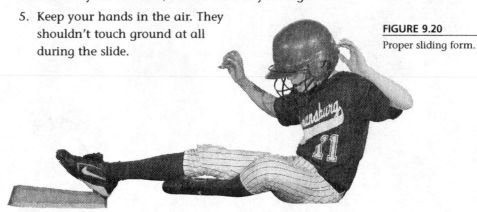

FIGURE 9.20
Proper sliding form.

Running from First to Second

The runner on first, while standing safely on first base, should look to the third base coach for any signal that a play—for example, a steal or hit-and-run—is on. Of course, such signs aren't necessary for teams in leagues in which leadoffs and this type of running are not allowed.

If the runner is in a league that doesn't allow leadoffs, he should get in a ready position to run, such as is shown in Figure 9.21.

If the runner is in a league that allows leadoffs and steals, he should take his lead after looking over at the third base coach. He

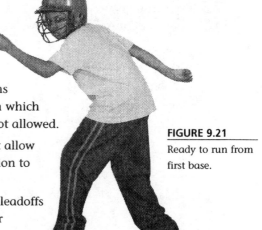

FIGURE 9.21
Ready to run from first base.

watches the pitcher as he takes his lead, always ready to quickly retreat to the base if the pitcher throws over.

After a pitcher delivers the ball, the runner's action is dictated by the play:

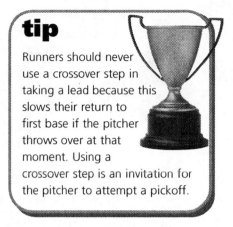

tip

Runners should never use a crossover step in taking a lead because this slows their return to first base if the pitcher throws over at that moment. Using a crossover step is an invitation for the pitcher to attempt a pickoff.

- **If the ball is caught by the catcher**—The runner should quickly return to first base, watching for a pickoff attempt from the catcher. Although the throw is farther than from the pitcher's mound, the runner's lead is longer (because he has taken his secondary lead), so he needs to get back to the base quickly.

- **If the ball is hit on the ground**—The runner should make a quick crossover step and run hard to second.

- **If the ball is hit on a line with less than two outs**—The runner shouldn't run until she's sure the ball is not going to be caught. After the ball gets through the infield, with no chance of being caught in the outfield, she should take off immediately for second base.

- **If the ball is hit in the air in the infield with less than two outs**—The runner should retreat to first base.

- **If the ball is hit in the air in the outfield with less than two outs**—The runner should go from one-third to halfway toward second, depending on the depth of the ball, unless his coach is telling him to tag up and advance after the catch. The runner goes as far as he can while still allowing enough time to retreat to first base if the ball is caught. If it is caught, he retreats immediately to first; if it drops, he takes off for second and looks to advance farther, watching his third base coach for guidance.

- **If there are two outs and the ball is hit anywhere in fair territory**—The runner should take off for second, running hard, even if it appears an out will be recorded. It's embarrassing when a baserunner is put out because his lack of hustle allowed the defense to make the play even though a fielder initially mishandled the ball.

Taking an Extra Base

Most kids love to run the bases, and they're more than happy to keep motoring as far as they can. So, they're naturally up to the task of taking an extra base—meaning going from first to third or from second to home on a single, or from first to home on a double. Although their enthusiasm is a great thing to see, it's greater to see it when they employ it wisely—that is, when they know when the time is right to take an extra base, and how to take it.

Let's look at two situations: when the runner begins on first base and when the runner begins on second base.

Runner on First Base

Crack! Andre hits a drive down the left field line, and Willie, on first, takes off for second, eyeing the play in front of him. He sees that the left fielder won't be able to retrieve the ball and throw him out at third, so he veers out slightly as he nears second, hits the inside of the bag with his left foot, and motors to third. The left fielder gets the ball into the infield, holding Andre to a single.

Now *that's* what you want to see. Following are the keys to a runner taking an extra base when he's on first.

As the runner advances toward second, he quickly assesses where the ball is headed and how far the outfielder has to run to retrieve it. If the runner sees he has a great chance to advance to third, he should veer out slightly as he nears second base, hit the inside of the bag (ideally with his left foot), and aggressively round the base (see Figure 9.22). As he rounds the base, he should pick up his third base coach for a verbal or visual signal to advance or stay. If the runner is advancing, he should take a quick look at his coach as he approaches third to see whether he should slide, come into the base standing up, or round third and continue home.

Balls hit to center or left field are easiest for the runner on first because she can track the play in front of her. However, she shouldn't keep looking at the ball or the fielders; she should just look long enough to know whether she should advance and

> **note**
>
> The base coaches are like traffic cops, directing traffic on the base paths. Coaches need to know when to send runners, when to hold them, and when to give runners their directions; runners need to be trained to receive those directions. The two most common errors of inexperienced coaches in this regard is giving no direction at all or giving it too late.

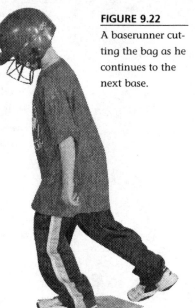

FIGURE 9.22
A baserunner cutting the bag as he continues to the next base.

always check with the third base coach as she rounds second. A runner should never look over her shoulder to see where the ball is after she's committed to going to third base because this slows her progress.

If the ball is hit to right-center or right field, the runner runs toward second, glancing at the ball as she does to get a feel for whether she can advance safely to third. As she approaches second base, she looks to her third base coach to see if she should continue to third. The coach should let the runner know as she's rounding second base whether she should advance, but if the coach gives no indication either way, the runner should decide based on what she saw developing as she neared second. If it would take a great throw, or two great throws, to get the runner at third, she should advance, but if she can be put out with an average play, she should stay at second.

> **note**
>
> The keys to knowing whether an extra base should be taken are how far the outfielder has to run to retrieve the ball, how many throws (one or two) have to be made, how deep the ball is hit, how good the fielders are, and how fast the runner is. You might not know specifically how good the fielders are, but you and the runner should know the other variables involved and make a good decision based on that information.

Runner on Second Base

One of the exciting plays in baseball is when a runner attempts to score from second on a single and the play is close at the plate. In an ideal world, the runner slides in, kicking up a cloud of dust, the umpire has a perfect view, and—if you are the coach of the team at bat—the umpire signals *safe*.

The keys to scoring from second base on a base hit are these:

- The runner gets a bigger lead off of second because it's harder to pick off a runner at that base than it is to pick him off at first base. So, the initial lead is longer and is lengthened by the secondary lead, taken after the pitcher begins his motion home.

- When the runner knows the ball is going to drop in the outfield, he runs hard to third base, looking at his third base coach, who signals him to either hold up at third or continue home. This sign should be given well before the runner gets to third, so he doesn't have to break his momentum if he does attempt to score.

- If the runner is waved home, he veers out slightly as he nears third, cuts the inside of the bag, and heads home as fast as he can. If the throw is coming from the right side of the field, the runner can steal a quick glance at the ball, but he shouldn't turn his head so much that his progress is slowed.

■ It's ideal that you train on-deck hitters to signal to runners coming home whether they should slide, but many youngsters forget this duty in the heat of the moment. So, this direction should, at least at the younger levels, be given by the third base coach. The runner should think "slide" and do so unless he's clearly directed to score standing up.

Running from Third to Home

When a runner is standing on third base, the third base coach should let him know what to do in various situations. As the pitcher prepares to pitch, the runner takes his lead off the base, standing in foul territory so any ball that hits him will be foul. If he stands in fair territory and is struck by a batted ball, he's out.

When the pitcher uses a windup, the runner can edge off the base a bit farther than if the pitcher is pitching from the stretch position. The runner should watch the pitch all the way in to the plate; often he can tell whether a pitch is going to be wild and can be ready to dash home if the pitch gets by the catcher.

However, the runner should have the weight on his right side as the pitch is coming in and be prepared to return to the bag after the pitch, if necessary.

With a runner on third, the third base coach instructs the runner in how to respond, given the situation:

■ **A ball hit in the air**—Start back to third base, unless there are two outs. Even with two outs, if a line drive is hit directly at an infielder (especially if it's the pitcher or third baseman), the runner should start back for third. Even if the ball is dropped,

note

Devise a set of hand signals to indicate plays or instructions to your hitters and baserunners. The third base coach usually flashes the signs. Make them simple enough that your players can remember them, but set up a system that the opponent can't easily decipher. For example, go through a series of signs before giving the "real" sign or make the "real" sign the third one in a series. Or have a wipe-off sign that is followed by the real sign.

Plays to signal include hit away, don't swing, bunt, steal, and hit-and-run.

tip

Although your runners should take their leads in fair territory, tell them to veer toward fair territory if the catcher is making a snap throw to try to catch them off base after the pitch. Runners shouldn't make their route to the bag longer, but when they return to the bag in fair territory, they make the throw from the catcher more difficult. Their bodies might shield the third baseman from the ball and thus cause an error.

the runner shouldn't try to advance if it's likely that the infielder can recover the ball in time and throw the runner out at home.

- **A ground ball with no outs or one out**—It depends on where the ball is hit and how deep the infielders are. If the infield is playing in and the ball is hit directly at an infielder, the runner should return to the bag. If the infield is back and the ball is hit deep or not directly at an infielder, the runner likely should go. If it's hit directly at the pitcher or third baseman, the runner should return to third. Often this determination is made by the third base coach before the play.

- **A ground ball hit with two outs**—The runner should, in most cases, go. The play will most likely be attempted at first base. One exception might be a dribbler in front of the plate that the catcher fields.

Above all else, the runner should listen to her third base coach, who will let her know what to do.

Stealing

Stealing bases is a great offensive weapon. If your league allows stealing, you should look to fully employ this strategy. But before you do, teach your players the skills involved in stealing. Speed is a great plus on a baserunner's side, but speed alone doesn't ensure the base will be stolen.

This section examines two scenarios: stealing second and stealing third.

Stealing Second

When a runner is safely on first, he looks to the third base coach for a sign. If the runner gets the sign to steal, he should not tip his hand to the defense by doing something he doesn't ordinarily do on first base. As usual, he takes his lead; watches the pitcher; and, when the time is right, uses a quick crossover step and takes off for second.

When is the time right? The simple answer is when the pitcher has committed to home plate—that is, he has begun his motion toward home and can't interrupt it without committing a balk.

Tell your players to watch a right-handed pitcher's heels to know when to go. If the pitcher's left heel lifts up, the pitcher is going home; if the right heel lifts up, the pitcher is attempting a pickoff.

note

Some coaches like to use a delayed steal. The runner doesn't break as a pitcher is delivering but breaks after the catcher has caught the pitch and has taken his eyes off the runner, assuming he won't go. As the catcher is easily tossing the ball back to the pitcher, the runner breaks for the next base. This tactic often catches the defense napping.

It's a little more difficult to time left-handed pitchers. Their right leg can be raised and they can still come to first base with the ball without committing to home plate. Base stealers have to make sure that a left-hander has committed to home before taking off.

Many pitchers use the same rhythm throughout a game. If they don't vary it with baserunners aboard, a savvy runner can time the rhythm and know when to go.

Timing is all-important in base stealing. Players with only average speed can be excellent base stealers if they can time their jump correctly. After they commit to running, their jump has as much to do with their success as their speed. They need to make a quick, powerful crossover step; stay low like a sprinter coming out of his blocks; and pump their arms as they sprint to second.

One quick glance at home plate, as the ball is reaching the catcher, is okay. The runner can pick up if the batter swings at the ball. If the batter hits a pop-up, of course, the runner has to scamper back to first base.

If a throw is coming to second, the runner should use a bent-leg slide into the bag.

> **note**
>
> Would-be base stealers have to keep their eyes on the pitcher and their ears tuned in to their first base coach. The coach will yell, "Back!" if the pitcher begins to throw over to first. This verbal instruction often saves the runner from being picked off.

Stealing Third

Stealing third is similar to stealing second, with these differences:

- The runner can get a bigger lead off second because the second baseman and shortstop can't hold the runner on (stand next to the base) like the first baseman does at first.

- Most steals of third are stolen off the pitcher, who often doesn't pay as close attention to a runner on second as he does to a runner on first. The runner on second can time the pitcher's rhythm and, armed with a bigger lead, often beat the throw to third, even though the throw for the catcher is a shorter one than the throw to second.

- Third base is easier to steal with a right-handed hitter batting because the catcher has to throw around the hitter.

These differences often make stealing third easier than stealing second. However, sometimes a steal of third is not necessarily a wise move. In general, you wouldn't want your players to attempt a steal of third if there are two outs. Why? Because the runner is already in scoring position and you hate to run yourself into the third out.

Many coaches also don't want to make the first out of an inning at third base because, if a runner is on second with no one out, there are three chances and many ways the runner can score.

Third base is most commonly stolen with one out because there are many ways a runner can score from third with one out (a ground out, a fly out, an infield single, a wild pitch, a passed ball, an error, a balk, and so on) that he can't score from second on. But that doesn't mean you can't go against the book once in a while and try a steal of third with no one out or two out!

Hit-and-Run

The hit-and-run is a strategy that attempts to advance the runner. The runner takes off as the pitcher delivers the pitch, much as in an attempted steal. It is best used with a hitter who can generally put his bat on the ball and an aware baserunner. The runner doesn't have to be fast, but she has to see the play developing and know how to respond.

The batter swings at the pitch whether it's a strike or a ball. Of course, if the batter is knocked down, it's a wild pitch, or it's so far out of the strike zone that he can't possibly reach it, the batter shouldn't swing, but he should swing at any pitch he can put his bat on. Why? Even swinging and missing is a greater distraction to the catcher than taking the pitch. The batter is trying to protect the runner, and hitting the ball does so. Swinging and missing does so to a lesser extent.

The ideal, of course, is to get a hit. On most hits, the runner can take an extra base because she was running on the pitch.

The runner's jump on the pitch is not quite as important in the hit-and-run as it is in the straight steal because the batter's job is to put his bat on the ball. The runner sneaks a look at the plate about the time the batter is swinging, ready to break back to the base if the batter pops the ball up in the infield or hits a ball in the outfield that is going to be caught. If the runner sees that the batter hasn't connected with the ball, she continues on to the base, attempting to steal it.

Tagging Up

A baserunner can touch his base after a ball is caught in the air and attempt to advance to the next base. Generally, this happens with a runner on second or third, or both, but at times a runner on first is able to tag up and advance to second on a deep fly ball as well.

The base coaches are instrumental here. When a ball is in the air and is likely to be caught by an outfielder and an advance after the catch is possible, the coach should instruct the runner to tag up. The runner retreats to the base, places a foot on it, and is in position to run hard to the next base after he sees the outfielder catch the ball. The runner watches the catch so he can get the best jump possible, rather than waiting to respond to the coach's verbal instruction to go.

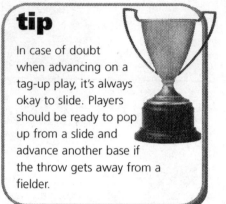

tip

In case of doubt when advancing on a tag-up play, it's always okay to slide. Players should be ready to pop up from a slide and advance another base if the throw gets away from a fielder.

When the catch is made, the runner pushes hard off the base and digs toward the next base. For runners going from second to third on a fly ball to right field or right-center, they shouldn't look back after they see the ball is caught; they should run for third and assume they are going to slide, unless the coach gives a "stand up" sign.

Likewise, for runners coming home, they can steal a peek at the ball if it's coming from the right side of the field, but if it's from left field or left-center, they need to run hard and assume they're sliding unless a coach or teammate tells them to stand up.

Common Errors in Baserunning

Here are common errors in baserunning and how to correct them:

- **The batter/runner slows as he nears first base, running to the base, not through it**—Remind the runner that he can run beyond the base and that he should not slow down until after he touches and passes the bag.

- **The runner slides on his side**—This results in scrapes and cuts. Help the runner learn the correct technique of sliding on the buttocks.

- **The runner slides with her hands down, scraping the ground**—This can both slow and injure the runner. Have her practice keeping her hands in the air as she slides. To emphasize this point, have her put her hands above her head as she begins her slide, although it doesn't matter where she keeps them, so long as they're not touching the ground.

- **The runner slows down in rounding a base or doesn't make a quick turn toward the next base**—The runner needs to cut the base by veering slightly to the outside of the bag as he approaches it and then touching the inside of the bag as he makes the turn for the next base.

- **The runner slows his progress on the base paths by continuing to look back at the ball**—A quick look at the ball is, in many cases, okay; repeated or prolonged looks are not. Instruct the runner to look at the ball as he is nearing a base, so he knows whether to advance, and then to focus on advancing.

- **The runner, about to attempt a steal, takes too long a leadoff and is picked off**—Encourage good leadoffs, but practice how far a runner can lead off and still get back to the base on a pickoff attempt. The extra 3" aren't worth being picked off for.

- **A fast runner is often thrown out in stolen-base attempts**—The runner needs to work on his timing and jump. He is likely not reading the pitcher well and either getting a late start or not making a strong crossover and driving hard to get immediately into top gear.

THE ABSOLUTE MINIMUM

This chapter covered the basic offensive skills of hitting, bunting, and baserunning, including the proper techniques for all the skills involved and common errors to watch for and correct. Among the key points to remember are

- No single batting stance is correct. Batters can use different stances, but help them find one in which they're comfortable, have correct body and bat position, and are ready to swing.

- The hitter's hands are at the top of the strike zone as he begins his swing.

- Timing is crucial in hitting, as is proper weight transfer from the back leg to the front leg. Coiling—closing the front shoulder, hip, and knee—prepares the batter to stride and swing.

- The batter keeps his weight on his back leg until he strides. The front foot stays closed during the stride; if it opens up toward the pitcher, the hips open up too soon and the batter loses power in his swing.

- When bunting, the barrel of the bat is angled up and the barrel begins at the top of the strike zone. The bunter holds the bat out in front of her body.

- The batter can either square around to bunt, with both feet nearly parallel to the pitcher, or pivot with the back foot.

- Drag bunts and push bunts are executed in hopes of getting base hits.

- The batter/runner runs hard *past* first base, not slowing until after he has touched the base.

- The runner takes a leadoff that he knows will not result in him being picked off the base.

continues

- The runner uses a bent-leg slide, sliding on the buttocks with her hands in air, when sliding into a base.

- The runner is ready to take an extra base and veers slightly to the outside of the bag as she approaches it and then touches the inside of the bag as she turns and advances to the next base.

- A base stealer needs to be able to read a pitcher; get a good jump; and use a strong, quick crossover step to begin his steal attempt. He stays low, drives his arms, and slides into the base.

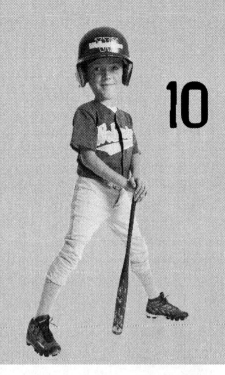

10

DEFENSIVE SKILLS AND TACTICS

Much of the glamour in baseball is focused on offense, but many games are won and lost at the youth level on defense. An average-at-best team on offense can excel, and even win league titles, if they play top-notch defense.

Topnotch defense doesn't mean shortstops are diving into the hole and throwing from their knees to nip the runner at first. It doesn't mean out-fielders are making spectacular, backs-to-the-plate, tumbling circus catches. It means your players know how to position themselves, know what play they need to make, and consistently execute the fundamentals (with the occasional outstanding play balanced out by the also occasional error).

It's too much to expect perfection from your players; even major leaguers make plenty of errors over the course of a season. But you can expect your players to know how to position themselves, to know what play to make, and to move toward more consistent execution of the fundamentals as the season progresses.

Of course, they need to be taught those fundamentals and learn the plays they need to make. This chapter helps you teach the basic defensive skills and tactics and know what to look for as you assess your players' progress.

Throwing

Being able to get zip on the ball is great, but it doesn't matter how fast a player can throw if he can't hit his target.

Here are the techniques to teach your players about throwing:

FIGURE 10.1
The proper grip.

- **Grip**—The player grips the ball with his fingertips (see Figure 10.1). The fingertips control the ball, not the palm. If the player holds the ball in his palm, the throw loses velocity and accuracy.

- **Front shoulder**—When the player has the ball, he turns his body so his front shoulder points to his target (see Figure 10.2).

- **Lead leg**—The lead leg is closer to the target. The thrower's body is sideways to the target (see Figure 10.2). Notice that the thrower's hips are closed to the target, just as a hitter's hips are closed to a pitcher before swinging.

- **Feet**—The back foot is perpendicular to the target, providing a base to push off of. The thrower pushes off this foot, stepping with his lead foot toward his target (see Figure 10.3).

- **Wrist**—As the thrower brings his arm back in preparation to throw, he cocks his wrist (see Figure 10.4). This provides leverage as the thrower brings his arm forward and releases the ball with a snap of the wrist.

- **Delivery**—The thrower uses a circular delivery, bringing the ball back and down behind his body and then up and over, releasing it as his hand continues across his body. The longer the throw, the longer the motion.

- **Follow-through**—The thrower follows through with his throwing arm down and in front of his body and his feet nearly parallel. His back leg will have swung around as his arm came overhead (see Figure 10.5).

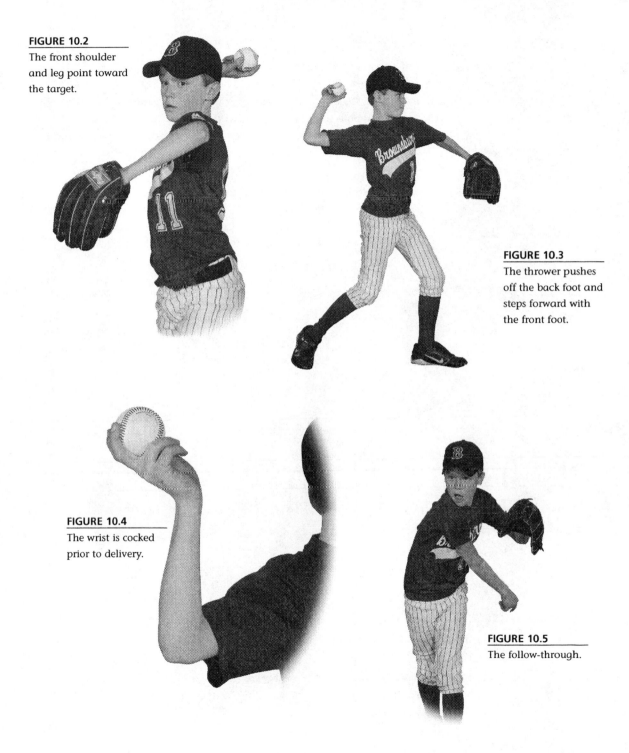

FIGURE 10.2
The front shoulder and leg point toward the target.

FIGURE 10.3
The thrower pushes off the back foot and steps forward with the front foot.

FIGURE 10.4
The wrist is cocked prior to delivery.

FIGURE 10.5
The follow-through.

Other Types of Throws

Your players should make overhand throws in almost all situations. At times you might see them make *sidearm throws*, slinging the ball to their target. Sidearm throws are hard to control. On occasion, a sidearm throw is the only choice, though, depending on from what angle the player is throwing, but it's rare that a sidearm throw will be called for. When you see your players dropping down and throwing three-quarter-arm or sidearm, steer them back to throwing overhand.

Another type of throw, one that is called for in close quarters (for example, a shortstop near the bag throwing to the second baseman for a force out) is the *snap throw*. The player uses a shorter motion with this throw, bringing the ball up only to his ear and extending his arm toward his target. The thrower's arm ends up parallel to the ground after following through. See Figures 10.6a–c for a snap throw.

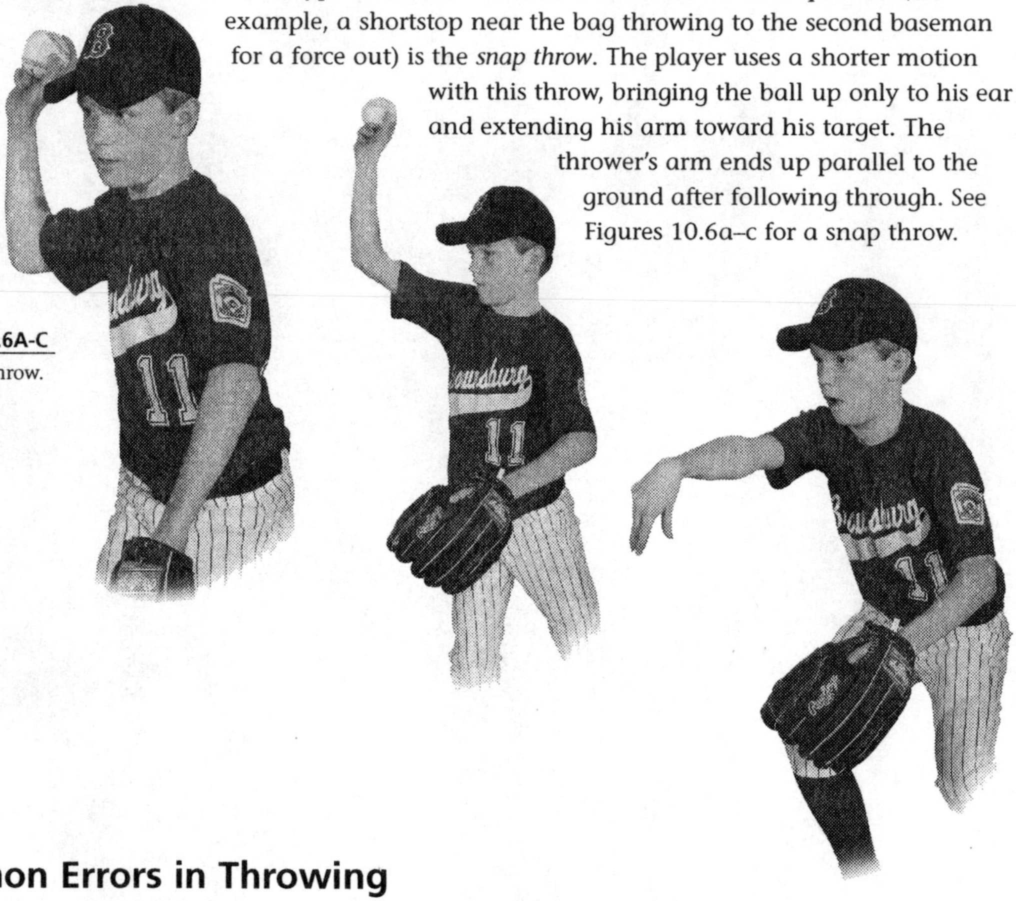

FIGURE 10.6A-C
The snap throw.

Common Errors in Throwing

Here are a couple of the common errors you might detect in throwing and how to correct them:

- **The thrower doesn't cock her wrist**—Throwing with a stiff wrist diminishes both velocity and accuracy. Have the player practice the cocking motion until it becomes natural.

■ **The thrower doesn't follow through completely**—A proper follow-through helps with both speed and accuracy. Demonstrate the proper follow-through, guide the player's arm through the motion, and have her practice that phase of the throw many times before practicing the entire throw.

Catching Throws

Catching throws is another fundamental defensive skill. Sometimes coaches, in their haste to get to other instruction, either skip or gloss over the techniques involved in catching throws. The techniques aren't complicated, but you need to teach them and make sure your players are developing them before you move on to more complicated skills.

In catching a ball thrown to him, a player should

1. Give his teammate a target to throw to—his open glove and throwing hand at chest level, with arms relaxed (see Figure 10.7).

2. Keep his eyes on the ball, all the way into the glove.

3. Go to the ball, moving as necessary if the ball is off target.

4. Give with the ball as it enters the glove, bending the elbows.

5. Squeeze the ball to make sure it doesn't drop out.

The glove angle depends on where the throw is. There are four situations you should teach here: catching above the waist, below the waist, to the side, and at chest level:

■ To catch a throw above the waist, the player's glove points up (see Figure 10.8).

■ To catch a throw below the waist, the player's glove points down (see Figure 10.9).

> **warning**
>
> Instruct your players to be ready to move when catching throws! Many kids expect thrown balls to come right to them, and they miss balls they could have caught because they don't move to catch the ball. Be sure they know their primary obligation is to catch the ball first. Then they can make whatever play they have.

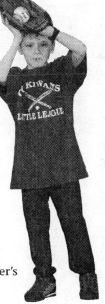

FIGURE 10.7
Catching a thrown ball.

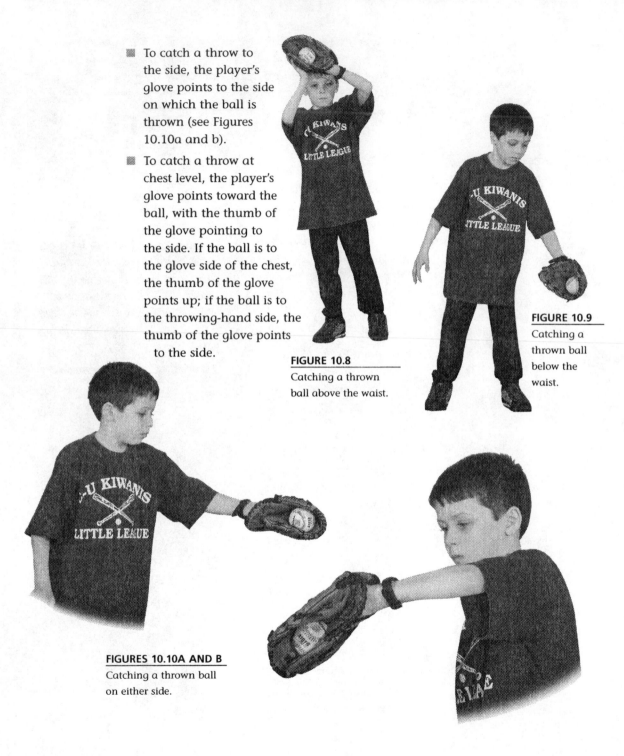

- To catch a throw to the side, the player's glove points to the side on which the ball is thrown (see Figures 10.10a and b).
- To catch a throw at chest level, the player's glove points toward the ball, with the thumb of the glove pointing to the side. If the ball is to the glove side of the chest, the thumb of the glove points up; if the ball is to the throwing-hand side, the thumb of the glove points to the side.

FIGURE 10.8
Catching a thrown ball above the waist.

FIGURE 10.9
Catching a thrown ball below the waist.

FIGURES 10.10A AND B
Catching a thrown ball on either side.

Common Errors in Catching

Here are some common errors players make when learning how to catch. Watch for them and use the suggested ways to correct them:

- **The player catching a throw isn't prepared to catch**—Remind her that she needs to be in the ready position, with her hands presenting a good target, before the throw is made. Have your assistant coach or a player throw grounders to you, with you completing the throw to her only when she demonstrates the ready position before you throw.

- **The player catching a throw doesn't move from his spot if the throw is off target**—Emphasize that the first duty is to catch the ball. Practice by making slightly off-target throws, making the player move to catch the ball.

- **The player catching a throw doesn't alter his approach to catching, whether the ball is above the waist or below the waist**—Work on each technique separately; then practice by interspersing high throws, low throws, and throws to the side.

Pitcher Skills

Just as hitting is a difficult skill to master, so is pitching. Many a coach has agonized over his pitcher's inability to find the plate. It takes years for good pitchers to develop all the skills involved, but you can help your pitchers develop by teaching them the correct techniques and working with them to find a smooth, efficient, and consistent delivery. This section helps you teach all the skills required of pitchers.

tip

For your pitchers, choose players who have strong and accurate arms. Accuracy is even more important than strength. Also choose players who *want* to pitch. Pitchers have to have some intestinal fortitude because they're in the spotlight. They also have to be able to deal with giving up some walks and hits.

Position on the Mound

For a kid who hasn't stood on a pitching mound before, it can be a foreign place. The mound is, of course, raised, and in the middle of it is a rubber slab that is a bit slippery. Complicating matters somewhat is that a pitcher needs to learn *two* positions on the mound: the position taken when pitching from a windup and that taken when pitching from the stretch position. Pitchers generally pitch from the stretch when runners are on base.

Position on the mound involves where a pitcher places his feet and where he places his glove and pitching hand. There are a variety of stances a pitcher can use on the mound. A pitcher might hold the ball in his glove anywhere from waist to chest height before starting his pitching motion, and he might stand on one end of the rubber, in the middle, or on the other end. He might stand with both feet on the rubber or with only one foot on it. All of these are okay. The most important thing is for pitchers to be comfortable on the mound and to approach their position in the same way each time.

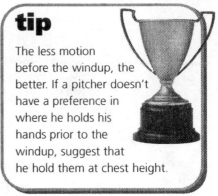

tip

The less motion before the windup, the better. If a pitcher doesn't have a preference in where he holds his hands prior to the windup, suggest that he hold them at chest height.

Grip

Two basic grips are with the seams (see Figure 10.11) and across the seams (see Figure 10.12). When gripping the ball with the seams, the ball tends to sink; when gripping it across the seams, it doesn't sink and can give the appearance of rising. What's important here is for the pitcher to use the grip that feels most comfortable.

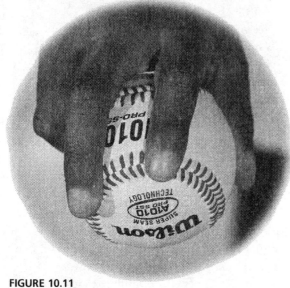

FIGURE 10.11
Gripping with
the seams.

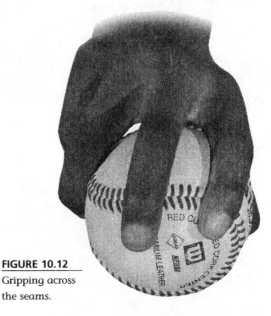

FIGURE 10.12
Gripping across
the seams.

Full Windup, Pivot, and Delivery

The windup begins with the right-handed pitcher taking a short step, moving his left foot to the side or behind the rubber (see Figure 10.13).

As the pitcher steps back, he moves his arms as well. A pitcher can bring his arms over his head as he begins to pivot on the rubber, or he can keep his arms at chest or waist level as he pivots.

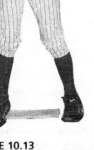

As the pitcher pivots, he pulls his lead leg up until the thigh is parallel to the ground or slightly higher, with the foot under the raised knee (see Figure 10.14). The pitching arm is behind the pitcher, down and toward second base. The back leg, planted on the rubber, is slightly flexed. The pitcher's body is closed to home plate.

The pitcher lowers his front leg and strides toward home plate as his hips open up toward the plate. This motion is propelled by the back leg pushing off the rubber. As this occurs, the arm comes forward in a circular motion. The stride is comfortable and propels the body forward but not so far that it is out of balance. The pitcher follows through with his back foot landing parallel to the front foot, in ready position to field (see Figure 10.15).

FIGURE 10.13
Beginning the pitching motion.

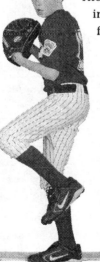

FIGURE 10.14
Leg kick, with the foot under the knee.

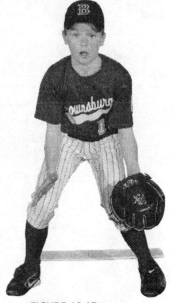

FIGURE 10.15
Following through into fielding position.

Pitching from the Stretch

When one or more runners are on base and stealing is allowed, pitchers typically pitch from the stretch position—meaning they *come set*, or pause, with their hands at their waist, before delivering the pitch (see Figure 10.16). This pause puts the brakes on runners who otherwise would have an easy time stealing a base.

From this set position, the pitcher lifts his leg, strides, and delivers the pitch.

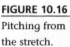

FIGURE 10.16
Pitching from the stretch.

> **warning**
>
> Don't allow your pitchers to throw curveballs or any pitch other than fastballs and change-ups. You can also protect their arms by not allowing them more than 75 pitches per game (or fewer, if that count is beyond your league's maximum).

Fielding the Position

Many young pitchers forget that they become another fielder as soon as they release the ball. Sometimes a pitcher's best friend can be his own glove.

The technique to follow through and end in good fielding position was already mentioned. Beyond that, pitchers need to be able to field bunts, cover first base on balls that pull the first baseman too far away from the bag, cover home on passed balls and wild pitches with a runner on third, and back up third base or home as needed. Here are technique tips for each skill:

- **Fielding bunts**—When a batter lays down a bunt, the pitcher springs off the mound, fields the ball cleanly, and makes the appropriate play. Common mistakes here include trying to pick up the ball too quickly or firing it without looking at the target. Instruct your pitchers to make sure they watch the ball into their gloves and make accurate throws.

- **Covering first base**—Teach your pitchers to break for first base on balls hit to the right side of the infield. If the first baseman is pulled away from the play, either in making a play on the ball or in trying to, the pitcher will have to take the throw from whoever fields the ball. The pitcher runs toward the first base line and, when he's about 20 feet from the base, cuts toward the bag (see Figure 10.17). With this angle, the pitcher has a better view of the throw coming toward him.

- **Covering home**—When the ball gets past the catcher and a runner is on third, the pitcher breaks to the plate to cover home. The pitcher prepares to take a throw and make a tag on the incoming runner.

■ **Backing up third or home**—When a throw is going either to third base or to home, the pitcher must back up the base to retrieve an overthrow. This can prevent a runner from taking an extra base.

FIGURE 10.17
Pitcher's route in covering first base.

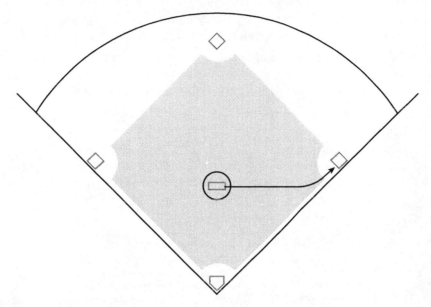

Keeping Baserunners Close

In leagues that permit leadoffs and steals, you have to teach your pitchers how to keep runners close by developing a good pickoff move. They can keep runners close by varying their rhythm when runners are on base (that is, varying the time they hold the ball in the set position before releasing it), by throwing to the base, and by stepping off the rubber. They shouldn't step off too often, however, because this disrupts their own rhythm as well.

Common Errors in Pitching

Common errors to watch for in pitching and ways to correct them include these:

■ **The pitcher isn't consistent in his positioning on the mound or in his delivery**—Consistency is critical in a pitcher's approach and delivery. Work with your pitcher to get smooth, efficient, and consistent mechanics.

■ **The pitcher takes too big a step back in beginning his windup**—This throws the pitcher's balance off. A short step back is all that's necessary. Work on shortening that phase of the delivery, putting a towel or something safe that the pitcher contacts if he steps too far back.

Catcher Skills

Catcher is one of the most demanding positions in baseball. Beyond the physical abilities associated with catching a ball, throwing it, and making all the requisite plays, the catcher often assumes a leadership role on the team. It's the catcher who works with the pitcher, helping him stay focused in crucial situations.

There's also more physical demand placed on the catcher than on other players. He has to squat for each pitch; wild pitches bounce off his body; baserunners trying to score slide into him at home plate. With all the gear a catcher wears, a catcher probably sweats more than other players, too, and this places further demand on the body.

Yet, some kids love to catch and have the physical and mental toughness that it takes to catch. In this section you're introduced to the basic skills of catching; through it, you should be able to help your young catchers develop.

Positioning

The catcher has two basic positions, one with no runners on base and one with a runner or runners on base.

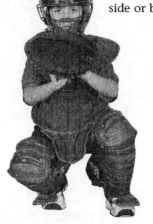

With no runners on base, the catcher gets in a comfortable crouch about two feet behind the plate, out of range of the batter's swing. He places his hand to his side or behind his back or glove to keep it from being hit by foul tips (see Figure 10.18). His feet are about shoulder-width apart and the weight is on the balls of his feet. The nonthrowing-side foot is slightly ahead of the other foot.

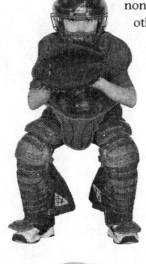

With one or more runners on base, the catcher assumes the "up" position, with the feet slightly wider apart than shoulder width and the rear end raised up a little higher (see Figure 10.19). This puts the catcher in position to get a throw off more quickly, should a runner attempt to steal.

FIGURE 10.18

Basic catching position with no one on base.

FIGURE 10.19

Catching position with a runner or runners on base.

Catching the Ball

The catcher gives the target to his pitcher before the pitcher begins his motion home. It's hard enough for the pitcher to hit a target when it's showing; it's that much harder to hit a location when the catcher doesn't show the pitcher where he wants the ball.

The catcher generally should give a low-strike target. Especially at younger levels, the target will be essentially the same throughout the game because pitchers don't have good enough control to nibble at corners.

For skilled pitchers at higher levels of youth play, a catcher might move his target around the strike zone. Let your catcher and pitcher know beforehand if you want them to try to hit the corners. If an outside or inside target is given, the catcher shifts his whole body, keeping the glove in the center of his body, rather than just shifting his glove. Instruct your catcher to move subtly, shortly before the pitcher delivers the ball, so the batter doesn't detect where the pitch is going.

Likewise, if a catcher sets up to receive a low strike down the center of the plate but the pitch is outside, he shifts his whole body, not just the glove, to catch the ball.

The catcher watches the pitch come in, moves to keep it as much as possible in the center of his body, and catches it. He doesn't push his glove forward to catch it, and he doesn't use his throwing hand to frame his glove, as other fielders do. These movements would invite injury to the catcher.

Blocking the Ball

One of the many skills a catcher needs to learn and refine is blocking pitches in the dirt with a runner or runners on base. Some pitches will come straight in but bounce before or after the plate; others will bounce to either side.

The catcher should be in the up position with runners on; this position helps because he's able to move more quickly than when he's squatting lower. In addition to positioning, a catcher can help himself by

- Reacting quickly to the ball and getting into position to block it
- Doing all he can, without putting himself in danger of being hit by a swung bat, to shorten the distance between himself and the where the ball will strike the ground
- Moving his whole body to the side to try to stay in front of the ball
- Dropping to the ground with his knees and closing off the open space between his legs by dropping his glove to the ground (see Figure 10.20)
- Leaning forward slightly and hunching the shoulders forward
- Trying to relax the body once in position, so the ball won't ricochet as far off a relaxed body

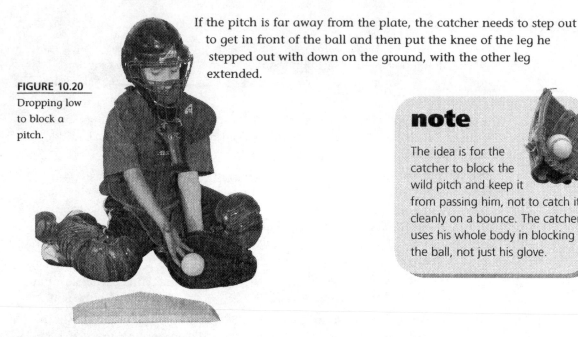

If the pitch is far away from the plate, the catcher needs to step out to get in front of the ball and then put the knee of the leg he stepped out with down on the ground, with the other leg extended.

FIGURE 10.20
Dropping low to block a pitch.

note

The idea is for the catcher to block the wild pitch and keep it from passing him, not to catch it cleanly on a bounce. The catcher uses his whole body in blocking the ball, not just his glove.

Throwing

In leagues that allow stealing, catchers must learn how to receive a pitch and quickly throw to a base. Teach your catchers to catch the ball and then pop up and close their hips by turning them to the bench on the first base side of the field (see Figure 10.21a). As they do, they rotate their shoulders perpendicular to the base they're throwing to and raise their glove hand near their ear. They grip the ball, take a step toward the base, and fire away, rotating their shoulders and following through (see Figure 10.21b).

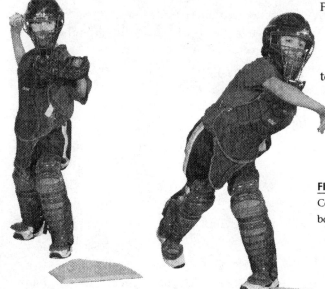

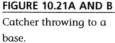

FIGURE 10.21A AND B
Catcher throwing to a base.

Catching Pop-ups

Catching a pop-up is harder for a catcher than it probably appears because in most cases a catcher is turning around and trying to locate the ball in foul territory. In addition, most pop-ups in the catcher's area tend to drift back toward the field, making it doubly hard because the catcher might find that he has to backtrack as the ball is coming down. And he's bogged down by his equipment, making it harder to move, and has his mask to deal with.

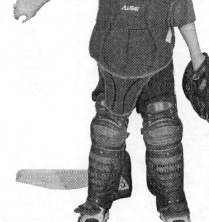

FIGURE 10.22
Catcher tosses his mask as he prepares to make a catch.

The three keys to a catcher catching a pop-up, then, are to

1. Locate the ball.
2. Get rid of the mask appropriately.
3. Make the catch.

The catcher takes his mask off immediately as he turns to locate the ball. He holds the mask in his hand until he knows where the ball is coming down and has gotten into position to catch it, or is nearly in position. He tosses the mask far enough away that he won't have a chance of stumbling over it, never taking his eyes off the ball (see Figure 10.22).

As the ball comes down and he's in position to catch it, he puts both hands about face height and watches the ball all the way into his glove (see Figure 10.23).

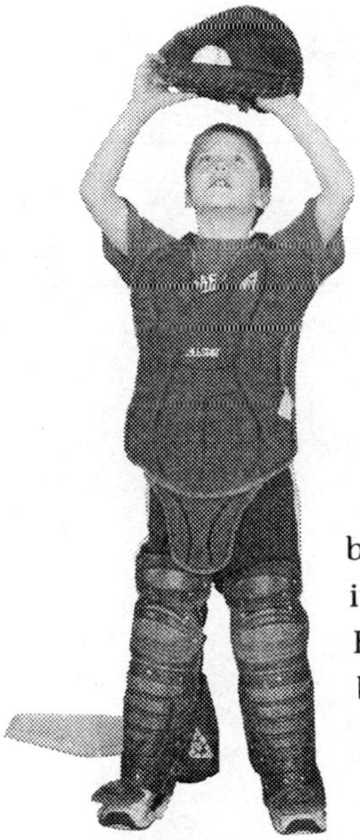

FIGURE 10.23
Catcher catching a pop-up.

Fielding Bunts and Slow Rollers

Your league might or might not allow bunts, but even if it doesn't, your catchers will have to be prepared to pop out from behind the plate, field a slow roller, and make an accurate throw to the proper base.

When fielding a bunt or slow roller, the catcher won't have time to take off his mask. He reacts to the ball as quickly as possible, popping out from behind the plate and using both hands to field the ball. As he goes to the ball, he gets his body in a position to make the throw to the proper base, if possible. That means that when he picks the ball up, he'll have his hips and shoulders perpendicular to the base he's throwing to, as opposed to squarely facing the base. Sometimes, of course, this won't be possible.

One of the trickier plays here is fielding a bunt or slow roller down the first base line. If it's close to the line, the catcher might have to field the ball and then take a step toward the middle of the infield before throwing to first base, to make sure his throw doesn't hit the runner.

Common Errors in Catching

Here are a few of the common errors in catching and ways to correct them:

- **The catcher doesn't use his body to block the ball but just tries to snare it with his glove**—Show the catcher how to protect his body and use it as a cushion to keep the ball in front of him. The object isn't to catch it, necessarily, but to block it. Throw pitches in the dirt to him and make the pitches progressively harder to handle as he builds his blocking skills.
- **The catcher trips over his mask in trying to catch a pop-up**—Help the catcher focus on "locate, go, throw"—locating the ball, going to where the ball will come down, and then throwing the mask.
- **The catcher makes poor throws after fielding bunts or slow rollers**—In haste, many catchers sling the ball sidearm after fielding a bunt or slow roller. Teach your catchers to throw overhand to the base.

Infielder Skills

Many players like to play the infield because a lot of action takes place there. Infielders need to be able to field ground balls and make accurate throws to the proper base. They also need to receive cutoff throws from the outfield, turn, and throw to the proper base. Earlier in the chapter you read about proper throwing technique. In this section you'll learn about

- The ready position
- Fielding grounders
- Holding runners on base
- Covering base on a steal attempt
- Tagging runners out
- Making force outs and double plays
- Executing rundowns
- Receiving throws from the outfield

Being in the Ready Position

Many times an infielder commits an error or doesn't reach a ball because he wasn't ready to react to the ball. Teach your infielders how to be ready for action before each pitch.

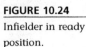

In the ready position, the infielder places his feet a little wider than shoulder-width apart, bends his knees, and places his weight on the balls of his feet (see Figure 10.24). His arms are in front of his body, but not so low to the ground that it's uncomfortable or makes it hard to get a quick start after the ball is hit. He holds his hands in a natural position, with the glove partially open to the hitter. As the pitcher delivers the ball, he is ready to move in any direction.

tip

Many youngsters think their glove has to be on or very near the ground and held wide open, facing the hitter. Teach them to hold their hands naturally, not too low or far from their bodies, and partially open. It's good to have the palms facing each other.

FIGURE 10.24

Infielder in ready position.

Fielding Ground Balls

From a good ready position, an infielder is ready to field a grounder and make the appropriate play. There are many types of ground balls: hard-hit balls, slow rollers, balls straight at the fielder, balls hit to the side, balls fielded on a short hop, and balls fielded on an in-between hop. Some balls stay low to the ground; others take high bounces.

As you practice infield play, hit many types of ground balls, not just those that are relatively soft and straight at the fielder. (Of course, especially for younger players, start with easier plays.)

Teach your infielders to charge the ball whenever possible. On hard-hit balls, they won't be able to do this, but the key is to get to the ball as quickly as possible while maintaining good position to cleanly field the ball and make the throw. By charging the ball, they are playing the ball, rather than sitting back and letting the ball play them. This has two advantages: They get to the ball more quickly, and they are in better position to field the ball. When they're back on their heels, it's very hard to field.

Let's look at the keys to fielding various types of ground balls.

Straight at the Fielder

In fielding grounders straight at them, your fielders should

1. Charge the ball.

2. Extend the arms in front of them and reach for the ball with the glove-side foot slightly forward (see Figure 10.25a).

3. Watch the ball into the glove, cushioning it with soft hands, and using the throwing hand as necessary to secure the ball in the glove (see Figure 10.25b).

4. Bring the glove up to the midsection and take the ball out.

5. Pivot, step toward the target, and use good throwing technique in throwing to the proper base (see Figure 10.25c).

FIGURE 10.25A–C

Fielding a straight-on ground ball.

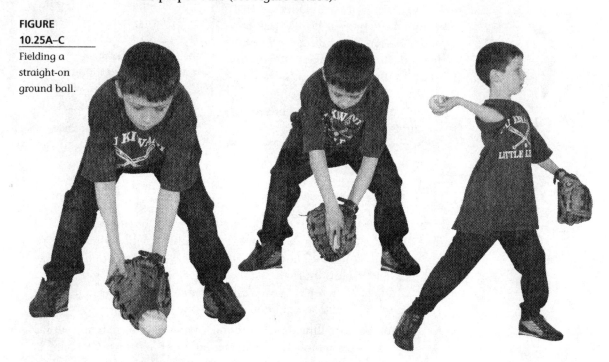

To the Side

Being in the ready position helps infielders be ready to move to either side to field a grounder. When a right-handed fielder moves to his left, he'll field the ball with an open glove, step toward the base, and make the throw (see Figures 10.26a and b). When a right-hander fields a ball to his right, if he has enough time, he can get in front of the ball and field it as he would if it were hit straight at him. If he doesn't have enough time to get in front of the ball, he'll have to backhand the ball, brake with his right foot to stop his momentum, and turn and throw to the proper base (see Figures 10.27a and b).

Occasionally, an infielder can backhand a ball and continue his momentum in the same direction as he makes the throw. For example, a first baseman or second baseman who backhands a ball and throws to the shortstop covering second base for a force out doesn't brake; he just continues toward second, making the throw as soon as he has control of the ball and his body and has a target to throw to.

**FIGURE
10.26A AND B**
Infielder fields a ball to his left and throws.

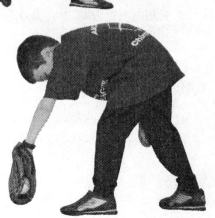

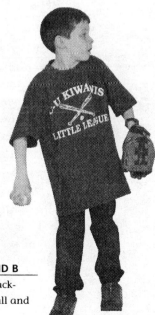

**FIGURE
10.27A AND B**
Infielder backhands a ball and throws.

Slow Rollers

Infielders have to be ready to charge slow rollers. A fielder uses mechanics similar to those used in fielding a ground ball hit straight at him, but an additional challenge with slow rollers is getting in good throwing position. The fielder's momentum often is carrying him away from his target. He must field the ball, quickly get into good throwing position, and make a strong overhand throw.

note

Emphasize the need to be in control before making a throw after fielding a slow roller. Teach fielders to field, plant, and throw overhand.

Holding Runners On

In leagues where stolen bases are allowed, your first baseman needs to know how to hold a runner on. This minimizes the lead a runner can safely take.

When a runner is on first base, the first baseman places his right foot on the side of the bag closest to home plate with his knees slightly bent. He extends his open glove toward the pitcher, ready to take a throw. When a throw is made, he quickly applies the tag. Generally, the tag is made low, close to the base, because this is the first point of contact for the baserunner's hand or foot in returning to the base.

When the pitch is made, the first baseman moves quickly to face home plate in good fielding position.

Covering Base on a Steal Attempt

On an attempted steal of second base, the second baseman normally covers the base when a right-handed hitter is up and the shortstop takes the throw when a left-handed hitter is hitting. This is because the infielders play most hitters to pull the ball—lefties to hit to the right side of the field and righties to hit to the left side.

Once your middle infielders (or the third baseman, on a steal attempt of third) see that the runner is attempting a steal, the infielder covering the base moves to the bag and prepares to take the throw, straddling the bag as he does and applying the tag.

tip

You might be able to teach older players to take a few shuffle steps toward the bag, with their bodies still squared to the plate, until the ball has passed the plate. That way, if the batter hits a ball in their direction, they still have a chance to field it. Once the ball passes the batter, the fielder quickly gets into position to receive the throw.

Tagging Runners Out

A tag play is in order any time a force situation is not. Tag situations include these:

- Runner on second
- Runner on third
- Runners on second and third
- Runners on first and third (the runner on third must be tagged, but the runner on first can be forced at second base)

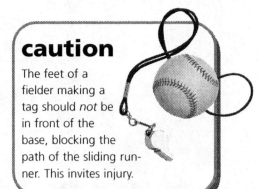

caution

The feet of a fielder making a tag should *not* be in front of the base, blocking the path of the sliding runner. This invites injury.

The runner must be tagged in those situations because he is not forced to advance; he advances on his own. When a runner does advance on his own, the fielder preparing to receive a throw for the tag play positions himself either with his feet straddling the base (see Figure 10.28a) or with his feet to the side of the base (see Figure 10.28b).

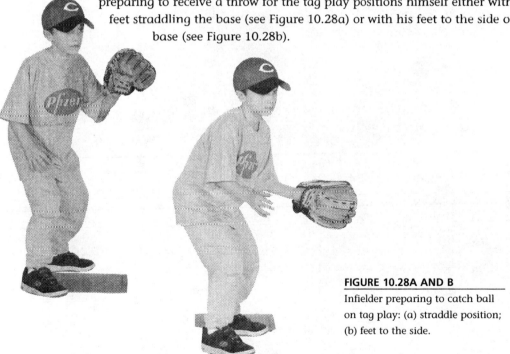

FIGURE 10.28A AND B
Infielder preparing to catch ball on tag play: (a) straddle position; (b) feet to the side.

The fielder presents a good target for his teammate to throw to, presenting a target about waist height. Players often try to throw the ball directly on the base; this is too difficult a throw and often makes it difficult for the receiver to catch the ball, even if it is on target, because the ball and the runner might be arriving at nearly the same spot at the same time.

As soon as the receiver catches the ball, he swiftly brings his glove down in front of the base and lets the sliding runner slide into the tag (see Figure 10.29). The fielder needs to be wary of the runner attempting to slide around the tag and position his glove appropriately, but in general, bringing the glove down directly in front of the base suffices.

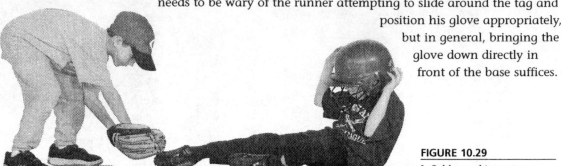

FIGURE 10.29
Infielder making a tag.

After the tag is made, the fielder scans the infield for any other potential plays on other baserunners.

Making Force Outs

Forces can occur at any base and be started by any infielder. Force situations include these: a runner on first, runners on first and second, bases loaded, and runners on first and third (the runner on first can be forced out at second base, but the runner on third is not forced to run).

Unless there are two outs and the easiest out is at first base, it's ideal to force out the lead runner. All your infielders will be involved in force plays, so practice all the variations many times, including the bases-loaded force at home.

The four crucial elements to making a force play are as follows:

caution

Many infielders, in their haste to make the force, take their eye off the ball and bobble it or miss it entirely. Caution your fielders to watch the ball into their gloves before making the throw.

- The fielder has to field the ball.
- The fielder has to make a good throw.
- The teammate receiving the throw has to get to the bag and be in good position to make the catch.
- The teammate has to make the catch and complete the force out.

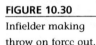

Throwing to Begin a Force Out

When the fielder has fielded the ball, he turns his shoulders and hips perpendicular to his target and makes the throw (see Figure 10.30). The throw comes in at chest height or slightly lower, so the fielder catching the ball can easily catch it.

Receiving the Throw

In receiving a throw on a force out, the fielder gets to the base as quickly as possible, places his left foot on the bag, and presents a target at chest height or slightly lower (see Figure 10.31).

Making the 3-1 Play

Your pitchers should be ready to cover first base on any ball hit to the right side of the infield. On occasion, even if the second baseman fields the ball, the first baseman will have made an attempt on the ball and will be too far out of position to get to the bag, so the pitcher has to hustle to the base and take the throw.

FIGURE 10.30
Infielder making throw on force out.

More common is the 3-1 play, with the first baseman fielding a ground ball and tossing it to the pitcher covering first. To make this play, the first baseman has to lead the pitcher with the toss, just like a quarterback leading his wide receiver. The pitcher shouldn't have to break stride as he catches the ball and steps on the base.

FIGURE 10.31
Infielder receiving a throw on a force out.

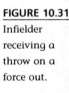

The pitcher catches the ball a step or two before he arrives at the bag (see Figure 10.32). If the throw arrives directly at the bag, the pitcher and baserunner have a greater chance of colliding, and the pitcher has a greater chance of missing the toss because he's concentrating on finding the base as well.

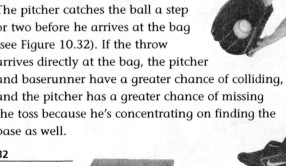

FIGURE 10.32
First baseman tosses to the pitcher for the force out.

Making Double Plays

Double plays are said to be a pitcher's best friend. They can rescue a pitcher from a jam and give the defense a lift, often swinging momentum from one team to the other. Sometimes single outs can be hard enough to come by; when a team gets two outs on one play, it can change the complexion of the game.

There are various double-play combinations: 6-4-3 (shortstop to second baseman to first baseman), 4-6-3, 5-4-3, 3-6-3, and 3-6-1, to name a few, though the latter play, with the pitcher covering first base and taking the throw from the shortstop, is a rare play in youth leagues. Following are technique tips for the second baseman and the shortstop in covering second on a double play attempt.

Second Baseman Covering Second

The second baseman covers second on a double play attempt when the ball is fielded by the third baseman or shortstop. When taking the throw to begin a double play, the second baseman has two choices in covering the bag:

tip

Coach your second baseman to run to the bag so the base is directly between him and the shortstop as the latter fields the ball to begin a double play. This makes the throw from the shortstop easier.

- He can cross over the bag on the shortstop side after receiving the throw, pivot, step toward first base, and throw (see Figures 10.33a and b).

- He can receive the throw; push off the back corner of the base with his left foot, moving him a step toward right field and out of the runner's way; step toward first base; and throw (see Figures 10.34a and b).

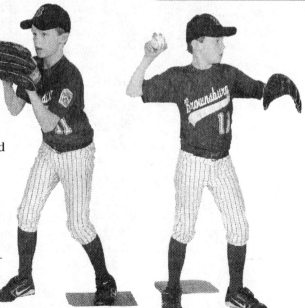

FIGURE 10.33A AND B
Second baseman crossing over the bag, pivoting, and throwing to first.

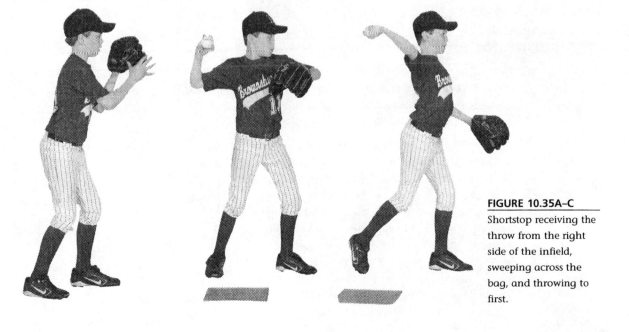

Shortstop Covering Second

The shortstop covers second base on any ball fielded on the right side of the infield or by the pitcher or catcher. Just as with the second baseman, the shortstop has two types of pivots he can make in this play.

On balls fielded by either the second baseman or first baseman, the shortstop moves to the base, straddles the back part of the base, receives the throw while sweeping the right foot across the base, and takes a step toward right field before stepping toward first base and throwing (see Figures 10.35a–c).

On balls fielded by the pitcher or catcher, the shortstop goes to the base, touches the inside part of the bag (closest to third base), receives the throw, takes a step toward third base, steps toward first, and throws (see Figures 10.36a–c).

FIGURE 10.34A AND B
Second baseman taking a step back, pivoting, and throwing to first.

FIGURE 10.35A–C
Shortstop receiving the throw from the right side of the infield, sweeping across the bag, and throwing to first.

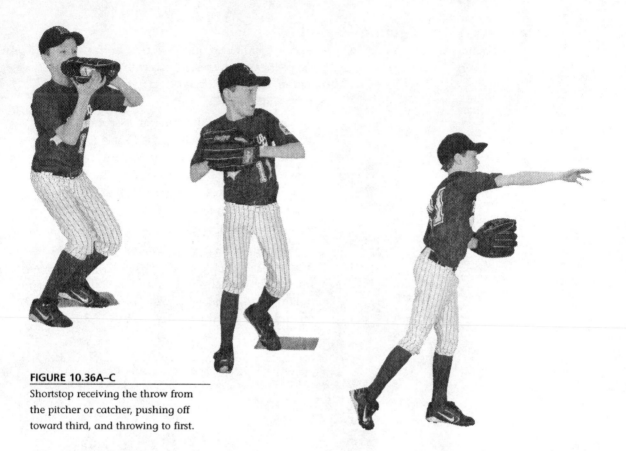

FIGURE 10.36A–C

Shortstop receiving the throw from the pitcher or catcher, pushing off toward third, and throwing to first.

Executing Rundowns

A rundown occurs when a baserunner is hung up between bases and is trying to move safely to one base or the other as two or more infielders are involved in the play, attempting to put him out.

The fielders are in charge on this play. The fielder with the ball holds the ball high, in a position ready to throw, and runs directly toward the runner, forcing the runner to commit to a direction. If the direction is toward the next base, the fielder throws the ball to her teammate covering that base. If this fielder cannot make a tag because the runner has reversed direction, the fielder holds the ball in a position ready to throw and runs the runner back to the previous base (see Figure 10.37).

tip

It's best to run a runner back to the previous base, rather than forward to the next base (for example, in a rundown between second and third, run the runner back to second, not forward to third). That way, if the runner manages to make it safely to the base, he will at least not advance a base.

The fielder throws the ball to her teammate covering the base, giving her teammate enough time to catch the ball and make the tag while not allowing the runner enough time to reverse direction and extend the play. The longer a play lasts and the more throws that are made, the more chances there are for a fielder to commit an error and allow the runner to safely reach base.

If it's executed correctly, only two or three players will handle the ball during a rundown, but all the infielders need to be prepared. The two infielders closest to the bases in which the runner is between are the two primary fielders, but the next closest fielders are backups.

For example, on a ground ball to the second baseman with a runner on second, the second baseman might fire the ball to the third baseman, with the runner stopping halfway between second and third. The second baseman

caution

The fielder should apply the tag with the ball held in the glove, not in the hand. The runner can easily jar the ball out of the hand.

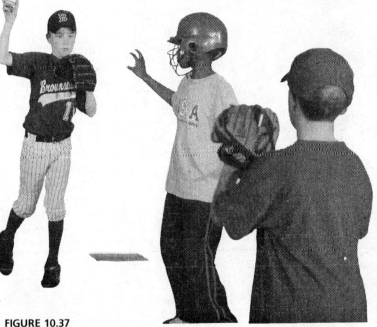

FIGURE 10.37
Infielders executing a rundown.

would then scamper over to cover second base, while the third baseman would run the runner back toward second. The shortstop would circle behind the third baseman and get in position to cover third base, in case the play went that far (which it shouldn't; the third baseman should run the runner back toward second and throw to the second baseman, and that player should make the putout).

You have a couple of options in teaching your players where to go after they make a throw during a rundown. One is to follow their throw—for example, a third baseman runs a runner back toward second and then throws to the second baseman as the runner nears second. The third baseman continues toward second, veering out of the path of the runner in case the runner turns and heads toward third. The third baseman would then get in position to receive any subsequent throws at second base; again, though, the ideal is to not have to make that many throws.

Another option is to have the third baseman in that same situation make the throw to the second baseman and then veer out of the baseline and peel back toward third, ready to back up the player who is covering third.

The keys in executing a rundown are to

1. Get the runner to commit to a direction.

2. Throw to the fielder covering the farthest base (for example, the third baseman in a rundown between second and third) to not allow the runner to advance to that base.

3. Have that fielder run the runner all the way back to the previous base, or to where the fielder's teammate can receive the throw and apply the tag.

4. Make the final throw with the right timing—enough time to apply the tag, but not so much time that the runner can stop and reverse his direction one more time.

Receiving Throws from the Outfield

Infielders act as cutoff players for hits in the outfield. As the outfielder fields the ball, the cutoff player lines himself up between the outfielder and the base the outfielder is throwing to, puts his arms up to help the outfielder easily see him, and receives the throw. He then turns and fires to the base, if necessary; his fellow infielders should be letting him know, as the outfielder's throw is in the air, which base to throw to or whether he should hold the ball. The cutoff player shouldn't just blindly wheel around and throw to a base. There might be no play on the runner going into that base, or the runner might have decided to stop at the previous base.

Cutoff duties generally are as follows:

- The shortstop is cutoff for throws from left and center fields.
- The second baseman is cutoff for throws from right field.
- The third baseman is cutoff for throws from left field to home.
- The first baseman is cutoff for throws from center field and right field to home.

Work with your outfielders and infielders in various cutoff situations, stressing good communication, proper alignment and depth of the fielders involved, and accurate throws. It's better to throw low and force your teammate to catch the ball on a bounce than to overthrow.

Common Errors in Infield Play

Some of the common errors in infield play include

- **The infielder is not in good ready position**—Sometimes players think that standing there watching the pitch makes them ready to field a ball. It doesn't. Teach your players what good ready position is and focus on this in practice.

- **The infielder doesn't charge the ball but lets the ball play him**—This results in lots of errors. Have drills in which infielders must charge balls hit to them.

- **The infielder doesn't get to the base quickly enough on a steal attempt**—Sometimes a fielder is too focused on the pitch to notice the baserunner. Teach good peripheral vision. The fielder who is charged with covering the base should watch the baserunner and be prepared to move to the base.

- **The infielder doesn't get into proper cutoff position**—Either the infielder forgets to get into position or goes too far into the outfield, shortening the outfielder's throw too much and making her own throw too far. Practice various cutoff plays in practice to give your players a feel for the positioning, communication, and throwing involved.

- **Infielders make too many throws during a rundown**—Practice this play and stress a minimum of throws: one, or, at most, two. Also stress running the runner back to the previous base.

Outfielder Skills

Outfielders need to be able to track down fly balls, catch them, field hits, make good throws to the infield, communicate well with teammates, and back each other up. This section explores the basic skills an outfielder needs to be successful.

Being in the Ready Position

The ready position is similar to that of an infielder's. Outfielders should bend their knees, feet a little more than shoulder-width apart; place their arms comfortably in front of them, glove waist high; and be focused on the hitter as the pitcher is delivering the pitch (see Figure 10.38). Their weight should be on the balls of their feet, ready to move in any direction.

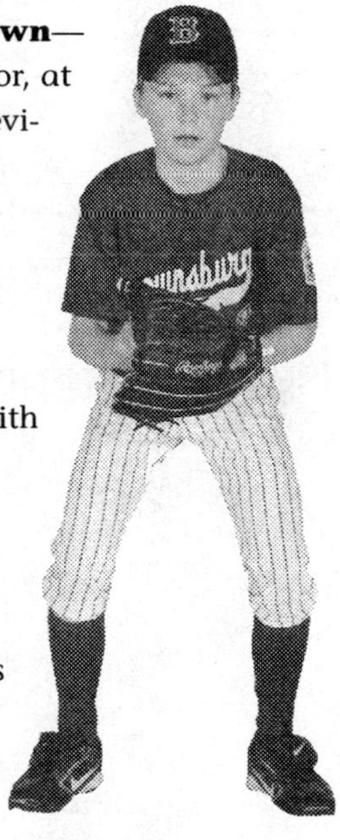

FIGURE 10.38

Outfielder in ready position.

Catching Fly Balls

One of the trickiest aspects of playing the outfield is judging fly balls. Many young-sters break in when a ball is hit because at the moment of contact, the ball is, of course, in front of them. Then they turn in dismay and track the ball down after it goes well over their heads. Conversely, some outfielders play it conservative and don't break in hard enough on fly balls hit in front of them, and they let balls drop in that they should have caught.

Judging fly balls takes a lot of practice. To judge fly balls and catch them, outfielders should

- Determine where the ball is going to land and run hard to that spot. This allows them time to adjust, if necessary.

- Run on the balls of their feet. Running on their heels makes the view of the ball shake; running on the balls of their feet keeps the view steady.

- Keep the ball in sight at all times.

- Keep their hands down as they run, until they're in position to make the catch.

- Position themselves behind the ball, so the play is in front of them, when possible. This is especially desirable with runners on base because the out-fielder's forward momentum will help her get more on her throw.

- Whenever possible, use two hands to catch the ball, catching it in front of the head (see Figure 10.39).

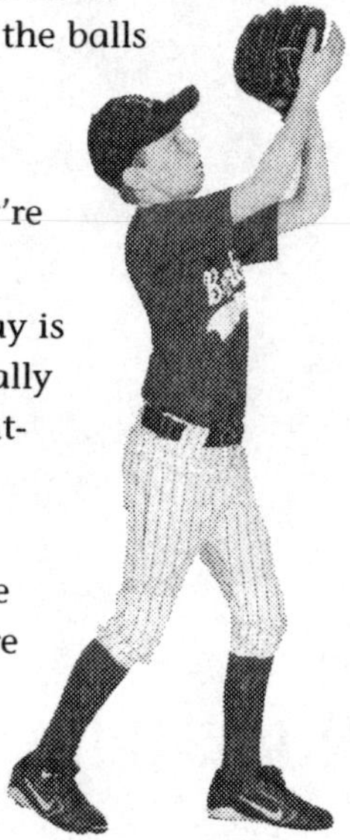

FIGURE 10.39
Outfielder catching fly ball with two hands.

Fielding Ground Balls

Outfielders have to field ground balls, too. The quicker they can get to them, the bet-ter. Just as with fly balls, they need to judge where the ball is going and run hard to that area, arriving there, if possible, so the ball is coming to them on their glove side. This helps them get more behind their throw. Fielding the ball on the glove side is especially important if the outfielder is trying to stop a baserunner from advanc-ing farther on the bases.

Most important, however, is for outfielders to cut off the ball before it gets past them. They need to get to the ball, watch it into the glove, and then quickly get into good throwing position, to throw to the proper infielder.

On balls hit on the ground directly in front of them, outfielders should charge the ball but not run so hard that they overrun the ball or can't field it cleanly.

Making Throws

Outfielders are required to make longer throws than infielders. Even with a cutoff player involved in the play, the outfielder generally makes the longer throw of the two.

To make strong, accurate throws, outfielders should keep the ball in front of them, whenever possible, to gain forward momentum toward the infield; they should use a crow hop, when appropriate, to add to that momentum; and they should throw overhand, concentrating on throwing on a line, and hopping the ball if necessary, rather than throwing a lollypop that floats high in the air.

What's a *crow hop*, and when should an outfielder use one? A crow hop is executed this way:

- A right-handed outfielder catches the ball with the glove-side foot (his left foot) slightly forward (see Figure 10.40a).
- He then brings his right foot forward with a quick hopping motion so it passes the left foot. He plants his right foot perpendicular to his target, rotating his shoulders perpendicular to his target as he does (see Figure 10.40b).
- The outfielder extends his throwing arm back, strides forward with the left leg, and throws as he shifts his weight forward (see Figure 10.40c).

As you teach this to your outfielders, you might help them remember the steps by saying, "Catch, hop, and throw." With the proper footwork, they'll gain power in their throws.

Outfielders should use a crow hop on a play in which they need to get the ball quickly into the infield and the play is in front of them. The outfielder should already be moving in the direction of his throw before he begins a crow hop.

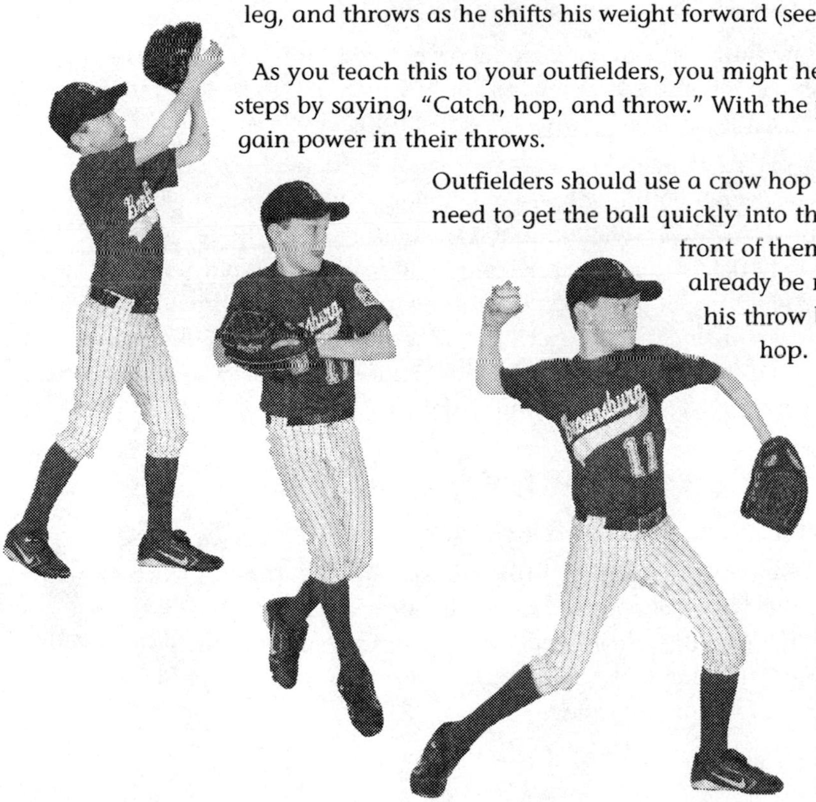

FIGURE 10.40A–C
Outfielder executing a crow hop. In (a), he catches the ball, left foot forward; in (b), he makes the hop; in (c) he strides and throws.

Communicating with and Backing Up Teammates

Communication is a vital aspect of playing the outfield. There are at least three things your outfielders should communicate to each other:

■ Whose ball it is

■ Where the ball is

■ Where to make the throw

Teach players to call any ball that is theirs if they are converging with another outfielder. They should yell, "I got it!" or "Mine!" as soon as they know they have the best shot at the ball. This helps avoid confusion and potential injury—as well as the embarrassment of both outfielders looking at each other and saying, "I thought *you* were going to get it."

Many times a fellow outfielder has a better view of the depth of the hit, and can yell "In!" or "Back!" to his teammate who is playing the ball. This is especially true for balls hit straight at an outfielder; these are hardest to judge.

Similarly, a fellow outfielder can see the play developing while his teammate is fielding the ball and can tell him "Second base!" or "Third base!" as he fields the ball. This helps the fielder know exactly where to go with the ball.

Also teach your players to back each other up. On a hit to left-center, the center fielder and left fielder are both involved—one making the play and the other running behind his teammate far enough that if the ball gets past, he can quickly retrieve it. The right fielder and center fielder play it similarly on plays in right-center, and the center fielder backs up both the right fielder and left fielder whenever possible, even when the ball is hit directly at the corner outfielder. If the ball goes over the head of the corner outfielder, the center fielder can often track it down more quickly if he runs hard from the beginning of the play to back up his teammate.

Common Errors in Playing the Outfield

Some of the common errors outfielders make, and ways to correct them, include

■ **They have trouble judging balls hit straight at them**—Teach them to stay put until they get a bead on the ball. Most of the time they'll break in and the ball goes over their heads. Teach teammates to also help them with the depth of the ball. Practice these types of hits to give your outfielders some experience in making this play.

- ■ **They don't communicate with their fellow outfielders**—Emphasize the need to communicate with each other and to clearly call the ball. Practice plays in which the outfielders are forced to call for the ball.

- ■ **They don't back each other up**—Often this translates into a single turning into a single and a two-base error, with the runner ending up on third. Two outfielders should be moving on each play in the outfield: one to make the play and the other to back up his teammate.

THE ABSOLUTE MINIMUM

This chapter focused on the skills your players need to develop to play good defense. Among the key points were

- ■ Pitchers need to be consistent on the mound in terms of their position on the rubber and their delivery.

- ■ Pitchers end their delivery in a position ready to field.

- ■ Catchers drop to their knees and drop their gloves to the ground as they prepare to block a pitch. They lean slightly forward and make their bodies soft, like a cushion, so the ball doesn't bounce far from them.

- ■ When a catcher goes after a pop-up, he takes off his mask, locates the ball, goes to where the ball will drop, and then tosses his mask a safe distance from him before making the catch.

- ■ Infielders watch ground balls into their gloves, charge the ball when possible, and make the throw to the appropriate base.

- ■ Outfielders run quickly to where they believe the fly ball will land, keep their eyes on the ball, and adjust as necessary as the ball comes down.

- ■ Outfielders use two hands whenever possible in catching a ball. They also try to keep the ball in front of them so their momentum is going forward when it's important to get the ball into the infield quickly.

- ■ Outfielders use a crow hop to gain power in their throws when they are moving to the ball in the direction of their throw.

- ■ Outfielders communicate clearly with each other and back each other up.

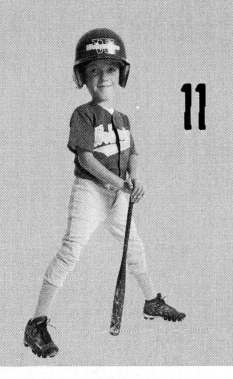

11

GAMES AND DRILLS

Now we get to what many coaches love: games and drills that will help their players improve their baseball abilities.

Use these 17 games as they are, adapt them to fit your needs, or use them to spur you on to creating your own games and drills. Know, too, that you can find many games elsewhere, including online. There is no lack of games out there. The challenge is to use games and drills that will benefit your players the most. Many games are boring, or make kids stand in line for a long time, or aren't realistic in terms of requiring kids to practice skills they will use in real contests. Steer clear of those types of games.

Instead, use games that put your players in game-like situations, that are fun, that call on them to execute the skills and tactics they will need to perform in real games, and that keep them active and not standing around waiting a long time for their turn.

Good luck in your season. Enjoy it, and help your players enjoy the great sport of baseball!

Infield Games

Here are seven games to use to practice a variety of infield defense—catcher defense, pitcher covering first, bunt defense, fielding grounders, making force outs and double plays, and communicating on pop-ups.

Game One

Name	Peg' em Out.
Purpose	To develop catchers' abilities to throw out base stealers.
Setup	Place a pitcher, catcher, first baseman, and second baseman or shortstop in position. Have three runners available to rotate stolen base attempts and fielders ready to rotate in as well (see Figure 11.1).
Description	As the pitcher pitches, the baserunner tries to steal and the catcher tries to throw him out. Rotate runners after each play.
Notes	Use your second catcher as well, rotating catchers. Give them equal attempts and see how many each can throw out. Also, you can place runners on first and second (along with a third baseman) and have the catcher choose which base to throw to.

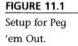

FIGURE 11.1
Setup for Peg 'em Out.

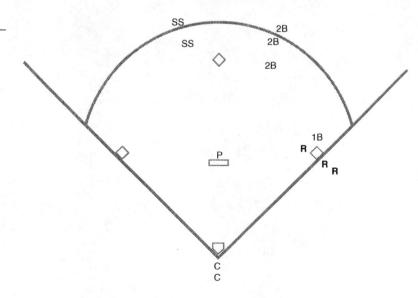

Game Two

Name	Dustbuster.
Purpose	To develop catchers' abilities to block pitches in the dirt.
Setup	Place a pitcher and catcher in position. A coach can be the pitcher.
Description	The pitcher pitches wild pitches and the catcher tries to block them, keeping the ball in front of him and not bouncing too far away.
Notes	Use whiffle balls to begin with; then advance to tennis balls and then regulation balls. Using the lighter, softer balls takes the fear away and helps the catcher focus on the proper techniques for blocking. Rotate two or more catchers, throwing 10 pitches to each and seeing how many each can successfully block. If your catchers are skilled, try this game with a baserunner on first and fielders at first and second base; the baserunner can try to advance to second at his own risk.

Game Three

Name	3 to 1.
Purpose	Develop the skill in pitchers of covering first base on ground balls hit to the right side.
Setup	Place a pitcher, first baseman, second baseman, and runner in position. (Have all pitchers line up near the mound, ready to take a turn. Also, have first baseman and second baseman be ready to rotate.) The runner stands in the batter's box, ready to run to first. The coach stands near home plate, ball in hand.

tip

In many of these games, we suggest that the coach roll or throw the ball to initiate play. You can also hit the ball to begin the play. The main thing is to get the ball where you want it to go. When the ball comes off the bat, it makes it more realistic for the kids, but it's sometimes harder to control. Begin the play in whatever way works best.

Description   The coach throws a ground ball to the right side, pulling the first baseman off the bag so that the pitcher has to cover first base (see Figure 11.2).

Notes   Rotate fielders on each play. The coach can throw so that sometimes the second baseman fields the ball. The main point is to make sure the first baseman is moving away from the bag, going after the ball, so the pitcher is forced to cover first.

FIGURE 11.2
Pitcher covers
first base in
3 to 1.

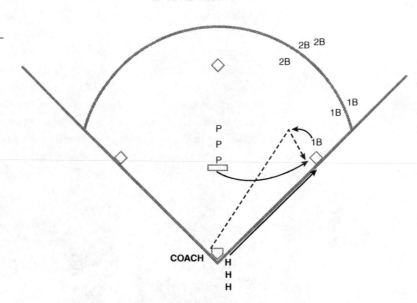

Game Four

Name   Bunt Defense.

Purpose   To develop the skills and instincts necessary to make the play on bunts.

Setup   Place an entire infield in position, with backups ready to rotate in. The coach stands near home plate, ball in hand. One or more runners can be placed on base.

Description   The coach rolls out bunts to various spots and the players make the appropriate play. Practice different situations—a runner on first, runners on first and third, or runners on first and second. And don't let players know where the ball is going.

Notes   It's always assumed there are no outs or one out. Rotate runners to keep the runners fresh.

Game Five

Name	Partner Rolls.
Purpose	To develop the fundamentals of fielding ground balls.
Setup	Pair up players. One player in each pair is on the back edge of the infield; the partner is about 20 feet away (see Figure 11.3).
Description	The player with the ball throws 10 grounders to his partner. The fielder fields the ball and makes an accurate throw back to his partner. They then switch roles, so the other player gets to field 10 grounders.
Notes	When the fielders can field grounders straight at them, vary this game by having the throwers throw ground balls to either side of the fielders.

FIGURE 11.3

Players paired up in Partner Rolls.

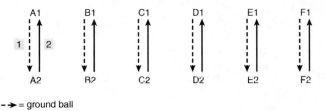

-- -> = ground ball
——> = throw

Game Six

Name	Force Feed.
Purpose	To develop the skills involved in making force plays and double plays.
Setup	Place an entire infield in position, with backups ready to rotate in. Place a runner on first base, on first and second, or on first and third. The coach stands near home plate, ball in hand.
Description	The coach throws ground balls on the infield in various spots; the players make the appropriate play at the appropriate base.
Notes	Begin with tosses straight at the infielders. As they improve, test them by making them go to their left or right. Rotate runners and fielders.

Game Seven

Name	Pop-up Drill.
Purpose	To develop reaction and communication skills and practice proper fundamentals on infield pop-ups.
Setup	Place an entire infield in place, with backups ready to rotate in. One coach stands between the mound and the third base line; the other coach stands between the mound and the first base line (see Figure 11.4).
Description	Have one coach toss pop-ups to the left side (third baseman and shortstop); have another coach toss to the right side (second baseman and first baseman). The players communicate with each other, call for the ball, and make the play.
Notes	You can involve outfielders as well, if you want, although they have a similar game designed for them.

FIGURE 11.4

Setup for Pop-up Drill.

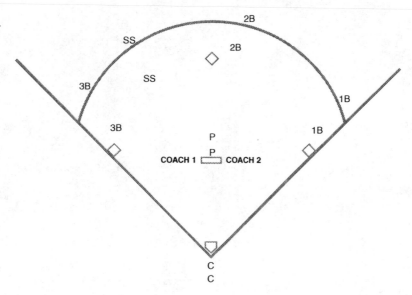

Outfield Games

Here are three games and drills to help your outfielders hone their skills. Outfielders also will be involved in the team defense games that follow this section.

Game One

Name	Drop Drill.
Purpose	To develop players' ability to react and move swiftly to fly balls.
Setup	Make two lines of players, with a coach ready to throw for each line (see Figure 11.5). Each coach has a ball.
Description	The first player in line faces the coach, about 15 feet away. The coach tosses the ball over the player's right shoulder. The player opens up his hips, runs under the ball, catches it, and throws it back to the coach.
Notes	You can vary the shoulder you're throwing over and the distance the ball goes. The key is for the player to get a good first step and open up his hips to run in the appropriate direction.

FIGURE 11.5

Setup and execution for Drop Drill.

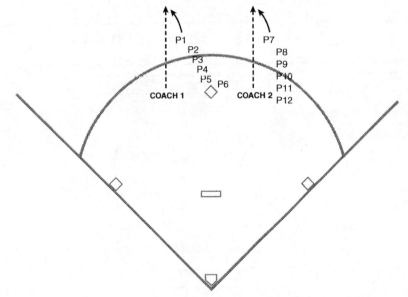

Game Two

Name	Bombs Away!
Purpose	To develop players' ability to catch balls on the run in the outfield.
Setup	Two coaches stand on either side of the pitching mound. The players are split into two groups.
Description	One player in each group runs toward her coach, flips him the ball, and continues running toward the outfield (see Figure 11.6). The coach tosses a fly ball for the player to run under, yelling "Ball!" as he does. The player then turns and looks for the ball, locates it, runs under it, catches it, and throws it back to the coach. The player then jogs back to the line as the next player begins his turn.

FIGURE 11.6

Executing the Bombs Away! game.

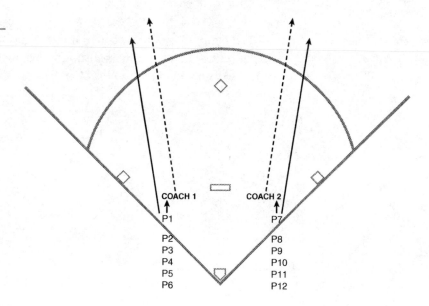

Game Three

Name	"Mine!"
Purpose	To help outfielders develop their communication skills.
Setup	Place two lines of outfielders in position (see Figure 11.7). The coach is near the shortstop area, ball in hand.

Description   The first two players in line are involved in the play. The coach tosses a fly ball between the two players. Based on where the ball is, one player calls "Mine!" while the other gives way and backs up his teammate. The player who catches the ball throws it to the coach, and the two players go to the end of their lines as the next two players move into position, ready to field.

Notes   Make sure the players not involved in the play give the two who are enough room.

FIGURE 11.7

Setup and play for "Mine!"

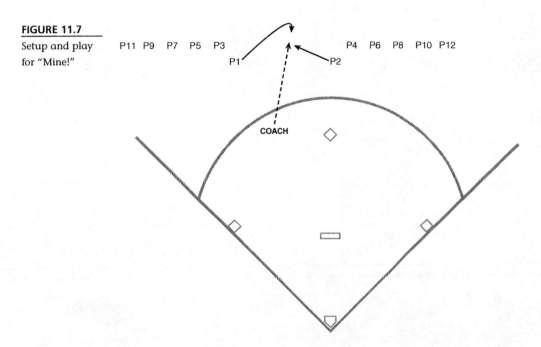

Team Defense Games

The following three games and drills work various aspects of the entire team defense. The games either focus on plays that involve the infield and the outfield working together, such as the Relay Drill, or help players practice skills that are necessary to execute in whatever position they're in, such as the Dive Drill and Make the Play.

Game One

Name	Dive Drill.
Purpose	To teach players how to dive properly, get up, and make a play.
Setup	Make two separate lines, one for outfield and one for infield. A different coach works with each line. Each line has a target player to throw to (see Figure 11.8).
Description	To begin, have the first player in each line start with the ball in his glove and kneeling on one knee. He dives, gets up, and throws to his target. The target player then throws the ball to the next player in line and the drill resumes.
Notes	As players progress, the coach can toss balls for the players, making them dive and make the throw to the target player.

FIGURE 11.8

Setup and execution for Dive Drill.

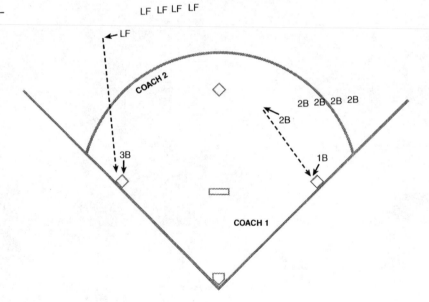

Game Two

Name	Make the Play.
Purpose	To develop good game smarts, making the best play available and working as a cohesive unit.
Setup	Place an entire team in the field (either a player or coach can pitch). The other players start out as hitters and baserunners.
Description	The pitcher soft-tosses and the hitter puts the ball in play. The defense tries to get the batter out.
Notes	Create different situations with one or more runners on base; with no outs, one out, or two outs; and so on. Switch hitters and runners with players in the field every 3–5 minutes.

Game Three

Name	Relay Drill.
Purpose	To practice all aspects of the relay: catching in the outfield; making the throw to the infielder; and (for the infield) proper positioning, catching, and throwing to the target.
Setup	Place three or four lines of players in position, as shown in Figure 11.9. Place players where you want them, depending on the play you are setting up.
Description	The coach tosses a ball to an outfielder, who catches and throws to the cutoff player, who turns and throws to the target.
Notes	Practice various setups, such as right fielder to second baseman to third baseman; left fielder to shortstop to catcher; and so on.
	To begin, you can run this play without baserunners. As fielders become more skilled, involve baserunners.
	There are five aspects of this play, as described in the purpose. Give instruction and feedback on all aspects. Points of emphasis for infielders include turning glove side when receiving the ball, catching it with two hands, and crow

hopping and throwing to the appropriate infielder's head (not his knees or right at the base because the ball tends to go in the dirt then).

FIGURE 11.9
One way to set up and execute Relay Drill.

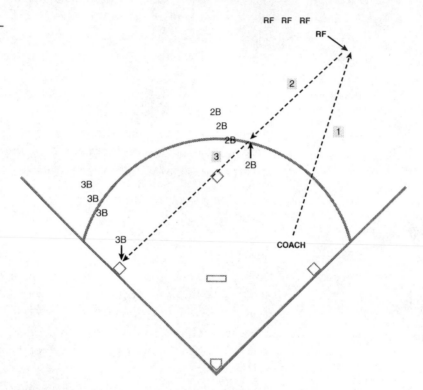

Hitting Games

Here are a couple of hitting games, one to practice hitting technique and the other to practice bunting skills.

Game One

Name	Short Toss.
Purpose	For hitters to practice their hitting form and going with the pitch.
Setup	The batter takes his stance at home plate. The coach stands 10–15 feet away and pitches from behind a screen.
Description	The coach pitches five pitches each to the inside part of the plate, outside part, and over the middle. The hitter focuses on good form and executes good swings, going with the

pitch and hitting outside pitches to the opposite field. The main focus is simply to get good cuts at the pitch. Hitters should use good judgment and not swing at bad pitches.

Notes   Mix the inside and outside pitches up to make it more challenging. If you don't have a screen, you can get a little farther away (for safety) and make the short tosses.

Game Two

Name   Bunt 'n Run.

Purpose   To develop bunting skills.

Setup   Place an entire infield in position. The coach can pitch, with a pitcher next to him, ready to field. A batter is in the batter's box, with other batters in line (see Figure 11.10).

Description   Have the batter lay down a bunt. Give each batter three bunt attempts; then rotate to the next batter.

Notes   First work on the bunting skills with no running involved. Later add the running for the batter. A bonus with this game is that it works defensive skills as well.

You can play 6-on-6. Have six batters bunt and see how many can either place good bunts or, if running, beat out bunts. Then switch the bunters with the fielders.

FIGURE 11.10
Setup for Bunt 'n Run.

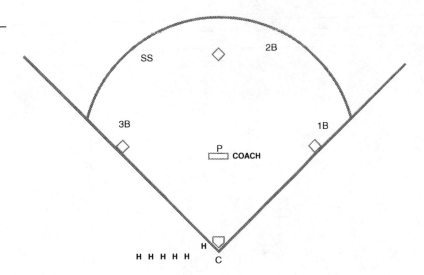

Baserunning Games

The following two games help develop baserunning skills. One develops the ability to round a base and go on to the next base, and the other helps kids develop the ability to tag up and advance on fly balls.

Game One

Name	Base Race.
Purpose	To develop the ability to go from first to third and from second to home by making good turns.
Setup	Place an even number of runners at each base (see Figure 11.11). The runners at each base constitute one team; there are four teams altogether.
Description	On the coach's command, one runner from each base takes off at the same time. They make a complete circuit of the bases (thus, the runner on second will end up at second, the runner on third will wind up at third, and so on). They tag hands with the next runner in line at their base, and that runner takes off. Whichever team completes the circuits first wins.
Notes	Focus on good baserunning skills, with the runners taking a banana turn, arcing out slightly as they near the base and then cutting the inside corner of the base with their left foot as they head for the next base.

FIGURE 11.11

Setup for Base Race.

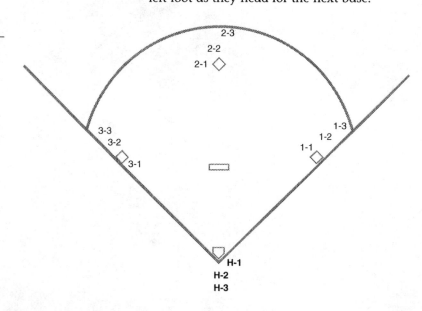

Game Two

Name	Tag-up Time!
Purpose	To help players learn to execute good baserunning skills in tag-up situations.
Setup	In the field, have a catcher, third baseman, and left fielder, and have a baserunner on third (see Figure 11.12). Have other runners lined up, ready to rotate in, and other outfielders ready to rotate in as well. After each play, the runner goes to the outfielder line, the third baseman goes to the runner line, and the outfielder becomes the third baseman. Have your assistant coach at third base in the coaching box.
Description	Hit fly balls to the left fielder. Make some shorter and some longer, and make the outfielder move. The coach instructs the runner to go or to stay, based on whether she believes the runner can score.
Notes	To make it fun, divide your players into two teams and keep track of how many runs they score. You can also try this with a runner or runners in different positions, or using a few more fielders.

FIGURE 11.12

Setup for
Tag-up Time!

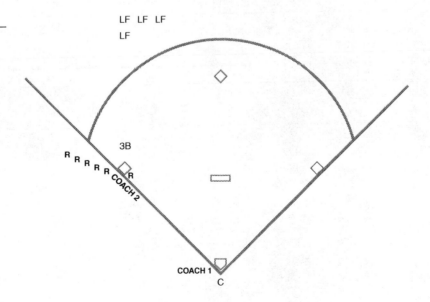

PART III

APPENDIXES

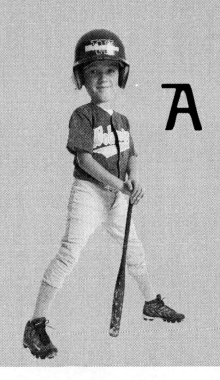

SAMPLE LETTER TO PARENTS

Note: This is a sample letter to parents of 6- and 7-year-olds. Your message to parents of older players would likely be a little different. Adjust the letter according to your needs, regardless of the age of your players.

Dear Parent(s):

I'm excited about the new season approaching, and I know you and your child are, too. I want to take a moment to introduce myself and let you know my approach to coaching.

I've been coaching for three years in the park district, beginning when my oldest son entered the league and am certified in first aid/CPR. Over the years, I've developed this coaching philosophy:

- The child is more important than winning. We will do our best to win, but helping each child develop his or her skills, learn more about baseball, and enjoy the experience—while providing for everyone's safety and well-being—take precedence over winning.

- Everyone gets equal playing time. Over the season, your child will play a variety of positions.

- We practice using games and drills that simulate what the players will experience in real games. We do this to practice skills and learn the rules of the game.

- I use positive reinforcement and plenty of encouragement as kids learn the skills. Baseball is a tough sport to master. My focus is to help players learn the fundamental skills and understand the basic rules and strategies of the sport.

What do I expect from the players? I expect them to show up to practice on time, to respect and listen to me, to respect their teammates, to try their hardest, and to have fun. I structure practices so the learning is fun.

What do I expect from parents? I expect them to

- Get their child to practices and games on time or to let me know if they're not coming

- Encourage and support their child and the team during games

- Refrain from booing or making negative remarks to the umpires or the other team

- Get involved in a variety of ways with the team (I'll fill you in at the first practice on these opportunities)

- Practice, if at all possible, with their child at home (I'll give you ideas for what to practice)

Please understand that baseball has some inherent risks. I enforce strict rules about the throwing of balls and the swinging of bats at practice, as well as the wearing of helmets. Even so, injuries can occur—generally minor, such as scrapes or bruises. I will do everything possible to run an injury-free practice, and I do know how to respond in case of an injury, but I do want you to know the chance of injury always exists in baseball, as in any other sport.

Our first practice is Monday, June 12, 5:30 p.m., at Blair Park. At that practice I will give you a full practice and game schedule. I will also give you a medical information sheet to fill out; this will let me know whether your child has any special medical conditions and who to contact in case of an emergency.

I'm eager for the season to start! See you on June 12.

In the meantime, feel free to contact me at 342-3537 before the first practice, or at any time during the season. Thanks for your attention to this letter, and I look forward to a great season coaching your child!

Sincerely,

[Name, phone number, address]

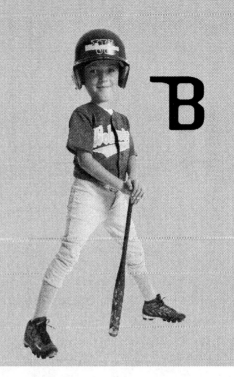

B

MEDICAL EMERGENCY FORM

Child's name _____ D.O.B. _____ Date _____

Address_____ Phone _____

IMPORTANT INFORMATION:

1. Does your child take daily medication? Yes ___ No ___

   If yes, please explain:

   _____

   _____

   _____

2. Does your child have any drug, food, or insect allergies? Yes ___ No ___

   If yes, please explain:

   _____

   _____

   _____

3. Does your child suffer from _____asthma, _____diabetes, or _____epilepsy? Check all that apply.

4. Will your child be bringing any medication to practices or games? Yes ___ No ___

   If yes, please name the medication and explain its purpose:

   _____

   _____

   _____

5. Has your child had a tetanus shot? Yes ___ No ___

6. Is there anything else pertinent regarding your child's health or physical condition? Is yes, please explain:

   _____

   _____

   _____

List two people to contact in case of an emergency:

Parent or guardian's name _____ Home phone_____

Address_____ Work phone_____

Second person's name _____ Home phone_____

Address_____ Work phone_____

Relationship to child _____

Family doctor _____ Phone_____

Family dentist _____ Phone_____

Health plan name _____

Health plan ID#_____

Parent or guardian's signature _____

Date _____

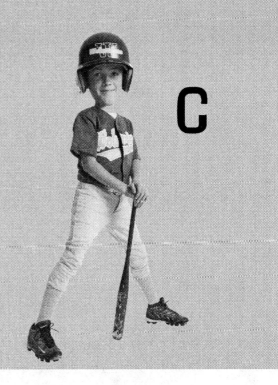

C

INJURY REPORT

Name of child: _____

Date: _____

Time: _____

Description of injury:

_____

_____

_____

_____

_____

_____

First aid administered:

_____

_____

_____

_____

_____

_____

Additional treatment administered:

_____

_____

_____

Referred to:

_____

_____

Signature of person administering first aid:

_____

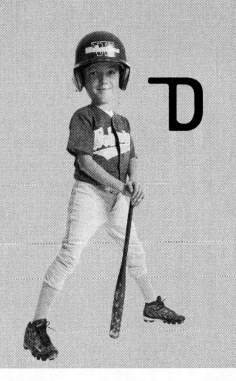

SEASON PLAN

Week	Purpose	Tactics/Skills	Rules
1			
2			
3			
4			
5			
6			
7			
8			

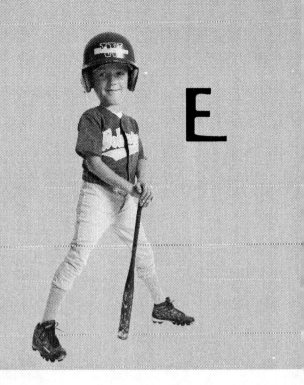

E

PRACTICE PLAN

Date _____ Place _____ Time _____

Equipment _____

Purpose _____

Activity	Description	Time	Comments
1. Warm-up			
2a. STATION 1: FIELDING			
2b. STATION 2: HITTING			

Activity	Description	Time	Comments
2c. STATION 3: BASERUNNING			
3. Wrap-up			

Notes:

_____

_____

_____

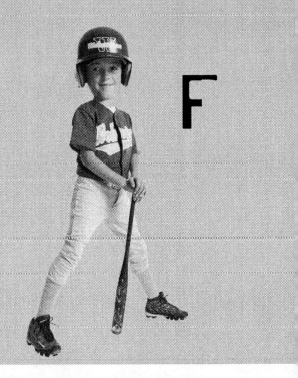

F

SEaSON EVALUATiON FORM

Note: Fill this out at season's end. Rate yourself honestly and use this form to note your areas of coaching excellence and areas for improvement for next season.

There are 14 main areas to consider. Respond to each statement made, scoring yourself between 1 and 5, based on this scale:

   1 = very poor

   2 = poor

   3 = average

   4 = good

   5 = very good

Note that similar statements will appear in more than one area; this is because the issue affects multiple areas.

1. Did Your Players Have Fun?

Statement	Rating: 1–5
The practice and playing environments were positive and enjoyable.	
I effectively organized practices.	
My players learned the skills they needed to be competitive.	
My players experienced individual successes in practices and games.	
I doled out playing time appropriately.	
I reinforced players' competence and helped them see positive aspects of their performance.	
I didn't overemphasize winning.	
Overall, I would say my players had fun playing baseball this season.	

2. Did Your Players Learn New Skills and Improve on Previously Learned Skills?

Statement	Rating: 1–5
My ability to teach skills enabled my players to learn what they needed to learn.	
I pushed player development of skills at an appropriate rate, neither too fast nor too slow.	
I helped all my players improve and didn't just focus on a certain set of players.	
I adjusted my teaching plan as necessary, according to the skill levels of my players.	
I planned and conducted practices effectively.	
I encouraged and supported my players as they continued their growth.	
Overall, I would say my players learned new skills and improved on any previously learned skills they came in with.	

3. Did You Help Your Players Understand the Game and Its Rules?

Statement	Rating: 1–5
I presented game-like situations for players in practice so they could gain a better understanding of how to respond to similar situations in games.	
I taught my players the appropriate rules and strategies of the game.	
My players showed, through their play, that they understood the basic rules and strategies.	
Overall, I would say I helped my players understand the rules and strategies of baseball.	

4. Did You Communicate Appropriately and Effectively?

Statement	Rating: 1–5
I let parents know my coaching philosophy before the season began.	
I let players and parents know what they could expect from me and what I expected from them.	
I communicated clearly with players, parents, umpires, other coaches, and league administrators.	
I kept parents informed and maintained a healthy flow of communication with them throughout the season.	
My players understood my skill instruction.	
My communications with my players were positive and authoritative.	
I was well-prepared for delivering the technical instruction my players needed.	
My players were prepared to respond appropriately in various game situations because I had prepared them for what they would encounter.	
My players paid attention to me when I spoke.	
My body language was in synch with my verbal messages.	
I was a good listener and focused on reading my players' body language and hearing and responding to their comments and questions.	
Overall, I would say I communicated appropriately and effectively with everyone involved.	

5. Did You Provide for Your Players' Safety?

Statement	Rating: 1–5
I was trained in CPR and first aid.	
I warned my players and their parents of the inherent risks of baseball.	
I had a well-stocked first aid kit on hand at practices and games and was prepared to use it.	
I knew of any allergies or other medical conditions of my players and how to respond regarding those conditions.	
I checked the practice and game fields for safety hazards and eliminated those hazards, if possible, before playing on the fields.	
I enforced rules regarding equipment use and player behavior that enhanced player safety.	
I provided proper supervision throughout each practice.	
I offered proper skill instruction so that players were prepared to play the positions I put them in.	
I took water breaks as appropriate during practice.	
I monitored my pitchers and allowed them a maximum of 75 pitches per game.	
Overall, I would say I adequately provided for my players' safety.	

6. Did You Plan and Conduct Effective Practices?

Statement	Rating: 1–5
Players paid attention to me because I had a purpose to what I was doing.	
There was no down time in practice while I was trying to figure out what to do next.	
Players were active and engaged at multiple stations that I ran simultaneously; they weren't standing around waiting for a turn.	
I used games and drills that were designed to teach a specific skill or tactic that I wanted my players to work on that day.	
My players learned new skills and refined ones they already had.	
My players had fun in practice.	
I had fun, too.	
Overall, I would say I adequately planned and conducted effective practices.	

7. Did Your Players Give Maximum Effort in Practices and Games?

Statement	Rating: 1–5
I didn't yell at players for errors and for their general quality of play.	
I didn't compare one player to another.	
I didn't create long lines in which players had to wait their turn.	
I taught players the skills they needed to know.	
I gave players specific technique goals to work toward.	
I provided specific, positive feedback.	
I encouraged my players, especially when they got down, and praised correct technique and effort.	
I genuinely cared for my players and let them know I cared about them and their achievements.	
I helped kids take home the positives of the practice or game.	
I praised hustle, desire, and teamwork shown in practices and games.	
I ran efficient, purposeful practices in which players were active and engaged the whole time.	
I valued each child for his or her own abilities and personality.	
I didn't play favorites with my players.	
I listened to my players.	
Overall, I would say my players gave maximum effort in practices and games.	

8. Did Your Players Leave the Games on the Field?

Statement	Rating: 1–5
I coached my players to keep the game in perspective—to give it their all but to let it go if they lost, and to not get a big head if they won.	
My players were not too high after a victory. They came back prepared to practice and play.	
My players were not too low after a loss. They came back prepared to practice and play.	
I talked appropriately with any of my players who were either too high or too low after a game, helping them to leave the game on the field.	
I talked appropriately with any of my players who had difficulty mastering his emotions on the field or immediately after a game. I steered the player toward mastering his emotions.	
I helped my players focus on the next game, regardless of the outcome.	
Overall, I would say my players left the games on the field.	

9. Did You Leave the Games on the Field?

Statement	Rating: 1–5
I didn't make too much out of a victory. I came back prepared to coach.	
I didn't get too low after a loss. I came back prepared to coach.	
I kept control of my emotions, win or lose.	
Overall, I would say I left the games on the field.	

10. Did You Conduct Yourself Appropriately?

Statement	Rating: 1–5
I communicated in positive ways with opposing coaches and players and with umpires.	
I coached within the rules and had my players play within them.	
I maintained control of my emotions in practices and games while providing the coaching and support my players needed.	
I kept the games in perspective and helped my players do the same.	
If I ever lost my cool, I admitted my mistake and apologized for it.	
I was an appropriate role model for my players.	
Overall, I would say I conducted myself appropriately as a coach.	

11. Did You Communicate Effectively with Parents and Involve Them in Positive Ways?

Statement	Rating: 1–5
I had few or no misunderstandings with parents regarding my coaching philosophy.	
I delegated responsibilities, sharing the workload with many parents and making my program stronger in the process.	
I wasn't as stressed as I might have been, had I not involved parents.	
I appropriately addressed the few misunderstandings or concerns parents had.	
Overall, I would say I communicated effectively with parents and involved them in positive ways.	

12. Did You Coach Appropriately During Games?

Statement	Rating: 1–5
I kept my strategy simple and based it on my players' strengths and abilities.	
I helped my players get mentally prepared for a game by focusing them on the fundamentals they needed to execute and on the game plan.	
I provided tactical direction and guidance throughout the game.	
I was encouraging and supportive.	
I gave technique tips and reminders and let the kids play, saving the error correction for the next practice.	
I tended to the kids' needs during the game—emotional and psychological as well as mental and physical.	
I helped players keep the game in proper perspective.	
I used a positive coaching approach.	
I effectively rotated players in and out.	
My players conducted themselves well during and after the game, including the post-game handshake.	
I held a brief post-game meeting, giving the kids some positives to take home, regardless of the outcome of the game.	
Overall, I would say I coached appropriately during games.	

13. Did You Win with Class and Lose with Dignity?

Statement	Rating: 1–5
I and my players shook hands with the other team, offering them congratulations.	
I thanked the umpires for volunteering their time.	
My team celebrated victories fully and in a way that showed respect for the other team.	
My players didn't hang their heads after a loss, no matter how hard the loss was.	
I helped the players regroup and take home positives from games we lost.	
Overall, I would say we won with class and lost with dignity.	

14. Did You Make the Experience Positive, Meaningful, and Fun for Your Players?

Statement	Rating: 1–5
My players still had the same zest and enthusiasm at the end of the season that they did at the beginning.	
My players seemed to want to come back for another season.	
My players learned the skills, tactics, and rules of the game.	
My players learned about themselves, learned what it means to be a member of a team, and grew up a bit.	
Overall, I would say the experience for my players was positive, meaningful, and fun.	

Index

How can we make this index more useful? Email us at indexes@quepublishing.com

open stance (hitting), 165

open substitution rules, 30

opponents, handling communication, 70

outfielders
backing up other fielders, 224
communication with other fielders, 224
crow hop throwing technique, 223
defensive skills, common errors, 224-225
drills
Bombs Away!, 234
Drop, 233
Mine!, 234-235
fair versus foul territory, 28
fly balls, catching, 222
ground balls, fielding, 222
qualities in, 221
ready position, 221
skills overview, 221
throwing to cutoff man, 220

outs
making on base paths, 39
scenarios, 33

over-coaching, signs of, 126

P - Q

parents
appropriate rules, 65
behavior during games, 64-65
child abuse, signs of, 68-69

coach communication with, 156
coaching advice, handling, 66
coaching from stands, 66
in-season communication issues, 63-64
inappropriate behavior, 66-68
involvement during games, 64-65
noncoaching roles, 98-99
preseason meetings, 62-63
yelling at children, 67-68
yelling at umpires, 67

Partner Rolls infield drill, 231

Peg'em Out infield drill, 228

physical development of players, 9

picking up the pitch (hitting), 166

pickoff moves, 42, 203

pinch hitting, position substitutions, 140

pitched balls, catcher blocking techniques, 205-206

pitchers
3-1 play with first baseman, 215
balks, 32, 40
ball delivery motion, 201-202
ball grips, 200
catchers, ball catching techniques, 205

fielding techniques, 202-203
common errors, 203
pickoff moves, 203
injury prevention, 79
inning restrictions, 32
pitch counts, 79
pitch types, caution against, 30
placement of, 30
position on mound, 199-200
qualities in, 199
skills overview, 199
starting age, 32
strike zone, 32
substitutions, 140

pitching
distances, 27
general rules, 31-32

pivoting (bunts), 174

placement of players, position guidelines, 31

planning
practices, 77
coaching instruction, 93-94
proper feedback, 93-94
safety issues, 92-93
simultaneous stations, 91-92
season, 88
adjusting for player ages, 89
purpose of, 88
rules, 89
sample 8-week plan, 89-90
sample 60-minute plan, 94
tactics and skills, 88

Do Even More
...In No Time

Get ready to cross off those items on your to-do list! *In No Time* helps you tackle the projects that you don't think you have time to finish. With shopping lists and step-by-step instructions, these books get you working toward accomplishing your goals.

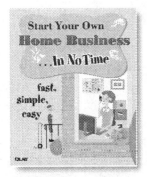

Start Your Own Home Business In No Time
ISBN: 0-7897-3224-6
$16.95

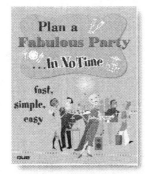

Plan a Fabulous Party In No Time
ISBN: 0-7897-3221-1
$16.95

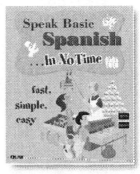

Speak Basic Spanish In No Time
ISBN: 0-7897-3223-8
$16.95

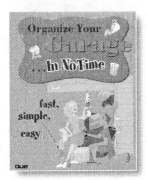

Organize Your Garage In No Time
ISBN: 0-7897-3219-X
$16.95

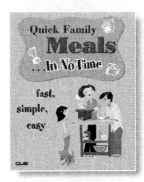

Quick Family Meals In No Time
ISBN: 0-7897-3299-8
$16.95

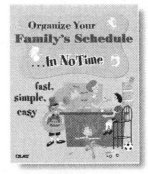

Organize Your Family's Schedule In No Time
ISBN: 0-7897-3220-3
$16.95

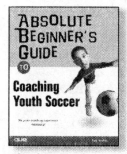
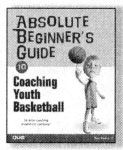
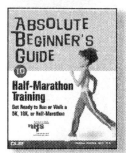
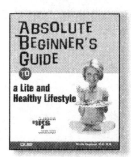
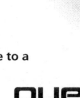